The Asthma Action Plan

About the author

John Chapman is an experienced practitioner in naturo-pathy, osteopathy, medical herbalism, homoeopathy and hypnotherapy with a clinic in Winchester in Hampshire, England. He has been over 20 years in full time practice and during this time has made a special study of asthma patients.

The

Asthma
Action Plan

John Chapman

N.D., D.O.

**Practical advice for gaining relief
from distressing symptoms**

Thorsons
An Imprint of HarperCollinsPublishers

To Jill for her patience, help
and friendship

Thorsons
An Imprint of HarperCollins*Publishers*
77–85 Fulham Palace Road,
Hammersmith, London W6 8JB
1160 Battery Street,
San Francisco, California 94111–1213

Published by Thorsons 1991
This edition 1993
1 3 5 7 9 10 8 6 4 2

© John Chapman 1991

John Chapman asserts the moral right to
be identified as the author of this work

A catalogue record for this book
is available from the British Library

ISBN 0 7225 2843 4

Printed in Great Britain by
Mackays of Chatham PLC, Kent

Contents

Introduction

When I was first invited to write this book, my first thought was to refuse on the grounds that any such work might be potentially dangerous to the health of certain individuals who followed the advice given instead of consulting a doctor. However, upon reflection I decided that most readers would be gifted with enough intelligence to seek the advice of their own medical practitioner before embarking on any self-help treatment that might aggravate their symptoms. This message is repeated at times throughout the book to remind the reader that we are dealing with a disease that is potentially a killer. It is a disease which costs the lives of over two thousand people each year in the UK alone.

None the less, there are a number of positive steps that may be taken towards alleviating some of the distressing symptoms of asthma. Before doing this, however, it would be wise as a first step to understand a little more of the disease and its various causes. I shall discuss this in chapter 1.

1
What is asthma?

Choking, gasping, heaving with the effort to obtain life-giving oxygen, he slowly began to choke on his own body fluids, as his lungs filled with mucus.

This is not the opening paragraph of a tense and thrilling novel: it is a description of an asthma sufferer in the throes of an acute attack. Over two thousand people die each year from asthma, and statistics show that it affects over 20 per cent of the population in one form or another.

Needless to say not every sufferer experiences this degree of an attack. For many, the condition is little more than a nuisance preventing them from participating in certain sports, or working at certain jobs. Some asthmatics have seasonal symptoms, either summer allergies from pollen or dust, or aggravations in the wet, cold winters. Most asthmatics will agree that their symptoms are generally worse at night. Why do sufferers experience their worst symptoms at night, or the early hours of the morning? In most cases it is due to the change in gravity: when the body is lying down, the air passages are somewhat narrower. Also, mucus is not excreted so easily from a person lying down, and so it can build up on the chest.

Another reason for some attacks at night is the allergy which some people have to the bed mite, to feather-filled pillows, or to house dust in general.

Although the onset of an attack is usually sudden, there often exist certain premonitory symptoms which can warn of the approach of an attack. These can be feelings of discomfort, or drowsiness, irritability, and depression of spirits. The patient can awaken in a state of great anxiety and alarm, with a sense of weight and tightness across the chest. Breathing comes with great difficulty and is accompanied by wheezing. The distress rapidly increases, and the patient can no longer retain the recumbent position, but gets up, and sits or stands with shoulders raised, head thrown back, and the whole body heaving with desperate efforts to breathe.

This presents a very disturbing picture, one not easily forgotten by loved ones who have nursed such symptoms through the night, or accompanied young babies in wailing ambulances to the nearest emergency unit for life-saving treatment.

Some only experience minor symptoms, but the condition nevertheless affects their lives. They may, for instance, when attempting to run or play some active sport, experience a tightness of the chest and an increasing difficulty in breathing the more they exert. This is relieved when they cease the activity and rest for a short while. Some may find that they must avoid certain atmospheres, for instance cigarette smoke in restricted spaces, or that certain weather conditions may cause some degree of discomfort in breathing. Misty or damp weather can be the worst culprits, and in some cases strong winds can literally take some people's breath away.

It may help at this point if we draw a mental picture of our lungs to refer to as we proceed through the book.

The lungs are very similar to an upside-down tree. The main trunk is called the *trachea*, which commences at the top of the throat. Halfway down the chest two branches appear, one going left and one right; these are a little narrower than the main trunk and are called *bronchi*.

From the two branches of the bronchi grow smaller and smaller branches, just as in a tree; these are called *bronchioles*. The two large branches with their multitude of smaller branches are enclosed in two delicate bags called lungs.

Let us now examine what happens within the lungs to cause such frightening and sometimes life-threatening symptoms.

At the commencement of an attack, a spasmodic contraction of the smaller bronchial tubes takes place. These are the smaller tubes leading off the main branches of the air passages, and a spasmodic contraction (a sudden narrowing) reduces the amount of air passing through them. The cause of this is variable and will be discussed later. It is this narrowing of the bronchial tubes, often accentuated by swelling of the epithelium lining (a delicate membranous covering inside the tubes), together with a marked increase in the production of mucus in the air passages, which is responsible for the great difficulty in breathing. This awful difficulty in drawing breath caused by the narrowing and the mucus produces the familiar wheezing noise, caused by air being forced through the narrowed passages, which is so characteristic of asthma.

Coughing is another characteristic symptom which often precedes or accompanies an asthmatic attack. The cough can be of two types: either a very loose cough with a great production of phlegm, due to the over-production of mucus in the bronchial tubes, or a very tight, dry cough produced by spasm in the bronchial tubes. Asthma can be divided into two broad categories called *extrinsic* and *intrinsic*.

Extrinsic, or allergic asthma

This is the most common form of asthma, and is caused by an allergic reaction within the body to certain things that most people do not react to.

This tendency to allergies is an inherited weakness which will be more thoroughly explored later in this book, but at this point I feel it would be useful to understand a little of what happens prior to and during an attack.

The immune system

Within each of us from birth is built a natural immune system, which works to protect us from harmful invaders. It has the ability to produce what are known as *antibodies*.

These antibodies are summoned by the immune system whenever an invader, such as a virus, enters the body. The antibodies then attack the invader and try to destroy it. During the process of attack and destroy, surface symptoms will often appear, such as a raised temperature or sweats, or the skin can change and produce rashes or spots. Observing these symptoms and the way they increase or decrease can often guide the person treating the illness as to which is winning: the invader or the antibodies.

In some people, however, the immune system goes wrong, and incorrectly summons the antibodies to attack. When this happens it is called an *allergic reaction*.

An *allergen* is anything which causes this allergic reaction to take place. It can vary from a food substance to a tree pollen or ordinary dust. When an allergen enters the system of an allergic person, it causes the immune system to manufacture special antibodies called *IgE antibodies*; these antibodies attach themselves to *mast cells* which occur in large numbers in our lungs and respiratory tubes.

When the IgE antibodies attach to the mast cells, a reaction takes place which causes the mast cells to release chemicals called *mediators*. Among these chemicals is *histamine*. These chemicals, when released by the body, cause a strong reaction within our lungs resulting in a tightening of the windpipes and a marked increase in the amount of mucus secreted by the delicate membranes which line them.

Intrinsic, or non-allergic asthma

This type of asthma does not respond to allergy triggers. It is caused by stress, infection, and environment such as weather, temperature, etc. Intrinsic asthma is more often found in weakened constitutions, particularly among those who have a history of lung conditions, such as bronchitis or pneumonia. The condition *diabetes mellitus* (diabetes) also produces a tendency toward asthma in some people, particularly elderly people. Intrinsic asthma is also more likely to be found among those who are over the age of thirty, while extrinsic asthma is common among those up to the age of thirty. This age line is of course not specific, and it must be remembered that extrinsic asthma can be found in older people just as intrinsic asthma can be found among young people.

Within these two categories of extrinsic and intrinsic will be found a number of different types of asthma, despite the similarity of the surface symptoms. Before embarking on any self-help programme it would be wise to try and understand which of the two categories your asthma comes into, as well as the form of asthma you suffer from. This will enable you to select the best self-help programme, or decide to enlist the aid of a practitioner qualified in one or more of the therapies outlined in this book. Let us now look at some of the different forms of asthma.

Bronchial asthma

A condition marked by recurrent attacks of *paroxysmal dyspnoea* (paroxysmal = spasm and *dyspnoea* = difficult or laboured breathing). This produces a wheezing due to spasmodic contraction of the bronchi (the larger air passages of the lungs). This is the most common form of asthma, which can be grouped under 'extrinsic'.

Bronchitic asthma

This is an asthma caused by an acute attack of bronchitis, an inflammatory condition of the mucous membrane which lines the bronchial tubes. Bronchitis is mostly caused by an infection. Bronchitic asthma is a common disease in the UK, due mainly to the damp and changeable climate. The condition can also arise as a result of inhaling irritating dust or vapours most common to industry, as well as heavy cigarette smoking or working in atmospheres polluted with smoke. This asthma comes under the heading 'intrinsic'. The terms 'bronchial' and 'bronchitic' asthma are often confused by the lay person but can be easily distinguished by remembering that bronchial asthma is extrinsic and bronchitic asthma is intrinsic.

Allergic asthma

This can often be caused by the presence of animals (particularly long-haired) or caged birds. Other common allergens include the house dust mite, the bed mite, house dust itself, and various kinds of pollens as well as moulds and fungi and their spores. At this point I think it worth mentioning that there are a number of drugs that if taken will cause or aggravate an asthma attack, among which are ibuprofen and aspirin or aspirin-based medicines.

It makes sense always to mention to your doctor, chemist or natural medicine practitioner that you suffer with asthma if requesting or receiving a prescription for medicines that have been prescribed for conditions not related to asthma.

Food asthma

This is also an allergic form of asthma except that the allergen is found in food. This includes yeast spores as well as the recognized additives used for colouring and preserving our food.

Recently, due to publicity, the larger manufacturers and retailers of food products have been making a point of selling foods without additives, whilst those with additives are being clearly labelled. Among the additives most likely to affect asthma are those with 'E' numbers – see the chapter on food and diet (chapter 8) for more information.

It is also possible that the condition *Candida albicans* might play a part in the food allergy reaction chain, as it is a condition which reacts to yeast spores.

Nervous asthma

The classical symptoms of bronchial asthma can be produced in some people by 'nerves'.

Fear or anxiety and their subsequent production of adrenalin can cause, in some people, an acute attack of 'asthma' which could become a serious life threat in some cases.

Cardiac asthma

This is an asthma that occurs in association with heart disease, such as left ventricle failure. In such cases it may be detrimental for the patient to attempt any of the self-help treatments outlined in this book without the full knowledge and co-operation of their doctor.

Pseudo asthma

This describes an asthma without pathological cause, that is to say without any underlying disease or allergic or nervous cause. Some environmental poisons may come under this heading as causative factors, as well as some osteopathic conditions which will be explained later in this book.

Extrinsic or intrinsic?

After many years of treating asthma I have come to realize that while it is important to diagnose the type of asthma in order to treat the fundamental cause, by its very nature asthma is a complex disease, and it is not always possible to divide it neatly into the two categories of extrinsic and intrinsic, because often both categories exist together in one person.

For example, if you take a case of chronic bronchitic asthma and examine the symptoms during an attack, you will note the presence of fear and anxiety, which are natural emotions when one is fighting for breath. It will also be noted that outside irritants will aggravate the condition – cigarette smoke, hairspray, fog, damp weather etc. And so within the original bronchitic asthma you have traces of nervous and allergic asthmas.

Likewise, you will find that a person who has suffered an early history as a child of recurring bronchitis will often develop a tendency in adulthood to allergic asthma as a result of the weakness laid down as a child.

When treating your asthma remember that the outside symptoms need to be taken into account and treated alongside the basic cause in order to speed the recovery.

For instance, if you were treating the asthma by diet, it would be wise to employ homoeopathic or herbal medicines at the same time in order to alleviate the symptoms of a possible attack during the period of treatment.

It would also be wise if treating, say, allergic asthma which has developed in a person who has a history of bronchitis as a child, to treat the constitution of the patient at the same time as the allergy in order to prevent a further manifestation of the weakness.

The asthma/eczema see-saw

It has long been accepted that some asthmatics also suffer from eczema, or that some eczema sufferers also have asthma. I have deliberately illustrated both sides of this coin, because frequently in the case of a child with asthma one or both parents are found to have a history of asthma or eczema or allergies in some degree. More often if you explore the family history, somewhere in a direct genetic line, often generations back, will be found a case of tuberculosis. In clinical practice I have found this link recurring often enough in cases of asthma or eczema to be of significance, and it is classed as the 'constitutional weakness' which underlies the asthma.

Sometimes a case of mild eczema in one parent will produce a baby with asthma tendencies, or asthma in the parent will produce eczema in the baby. The chances of a baby being born with one of these conditions is greatly increased if both parents have the weakness. Likewise, it is quite rare for a child to have asthma if there is no family weakness.

The see-saw

In cases where both conditions exist in the body it will normally be found that only one is prevalent. For instance, when the eczema is particularly troublesome it will be found that the asthma is either very mild or nonexistent. Likewise if the asthma is troublesome, the eczema is mild or nonexistent.

This phenomenon is known as the asthma/eczema see-saw and was recognized by Dr Samuel Hahnemann, who was born in Meissen, Germany in 1755. He formulated a basic philosophy of disease in which he states that all men and women were born with basic weaknesses already present in the body. These weaknesses arose from inherited genetic trends developed over hundreds of years, the results of the rampant diseases which swept the world, such as tuberculosis, gonorrhoea, and syphilis. These and other diseases took their toll in human life, but those who survived paid a price, and eventually passed on to their children and their children's children weaknesses which manifested in various forms. Although in this century we have conquered these diseases, they are still rampant in the Third World and their effects can be seen today.

The genetic weaknesses, much diluted with each generation that has passed, have now become intermixed and these *miasms*, as Hahnemann called them, exist within each of us although only one usually predominates.

The constitutional weakness

The broad approach to the effective treatment of asthma adopted by practitioners of alternative medicine acknowledges the presence of the miasms and seeks to identify and treat the predominating one. They can manifest in different ways: for instance, the gonorrhoea miasm can surface generations later in the form of chronic arthritis, whilst the tubercular miasm most often surfaces in the form of asthma or eczema.

The Natural Medicine practitioner will go to great lengths to avoid suppressing either the asthma or the eczema condition, for by doing so you are inviting a more chronic condition to develop. This is illustrated by the use of cortisone-based creams employed by the medical orthodoxy to treat eczema, the skin will improve with their use, but often at the expense of the asthma which flares up. When the asthma is then treated with one of the frequently prescribed inhalers, it will alleviate the asthma but the eczema comes back. You will see from this illustration why many cases of asthma/eczema are never cured.

This is where the division between alternative and orthodox medicine becomes most apparent: the former attempts to treat the cause, whilst the latter appears to have slipped into the habit of treating the symptoms.

Drugs used in asthma

I do not intend to deride the methods of treatment used by orthodoxy for asthma – many people owe their lives to the drugs regularly prescribed by their doctor. Unfortunately many of the drugs used today, although very sophisticated, do have side-effects, and as already stated, do not produce the cure.

The drugs used in asthma today fall broadly into three categories: *bronchodilators; mast cell stabilizers* and *corticosteroids.*

Bronchodilators act by relaxing the muscles surrounding the bronchioles (the smaller tubes of the lungs).

Mast cell stabilizers act by preventing the release from

certain cells in the body of strong chemicals known as *mediators* (see page 12).

Corticosteroids act by reducing the inflammation, either in the nasal or bronchial passages.

The bronchodilators themselves fall into three categories known as *sympathomimetics*, *anticholinergics* and *xanthines*.

Sympathomimetic and anticholinergic drugs produce their relaxing effect on the bronchioles by interfering with nerve signals passed to the muscles through the nervous system.

Xanthine drugs are thought to relax the muscles in the bronchioles by a direct effect on the muscle fibre, but their precise action is not known.

The benefit of the bronchodilators is usually to improve breathing within a few minutes, but often repeated doses are needed to maintain the improvement.

Side-effects

Side-effects of sympathomimetic drugs can include palpitations (rapid action of the heart), and trembling.

Side-effects of anticholinergic drugs can include dry mouth, blurred vision, and difficulty in passing urine.

Side-effects of xanthine drugs may include headaches or nausea.

Sympathomimetic and xanthine drugs should be taken with caution by those with heart problems, high blood pressure, or an overactive thyroid gland.

Anticholinergic drugs should be taken with caution by those with urinary retention or a tendency to glaucoma.

Examples of drugs

Bronchodilators

Sympathomimetics
Isoprenaline Brand names include Iso-autohaler, Medihaler-iso, Medihaler-duo, Saventrine, and Intal-compound.
Salbutamol Brand names include Ventolin, Salbulin, aerolin and Cobutalin.

Anticholinergics
Atropine, because of its antispasmodic properties, is used for many conditions. Most people will recognize it as a

treatment for enlarging the pupil of the eye. When used as a bronchodilator it is usually in the form of an inhaler with other drugs.

Xanthines

Theophylline Brand names include Lasma, Nuelin, Phyllocontin, Sabidal SR, Franol and Tedral.

Treatment with this drug should be monitored by the prescribing doctor because the effective dose is very close to the toxic dose. Special precautions should be observed by those with long-term liver problems, angina, or gastrointestinal ulcers; smokers; pregnant and breast-feeding women.

Most bronchodilators are inhaled directly into the lungs by the use of an inhaler, or 'puffer', an insufflation cartridge, or a nebulizer.

Mast cell stabilizers

Sodium cromoglycate Brand names include Intal, Nalcrom, Opticrom and Rynacrom.

Corticosteroids

Beclomethasone Brand names include Becloforte, Beconase, Becotide, Propaderm, Propaderm A and Ventide. This drug is used mostly for people whose asthma does not respond to bronchodilators alone.

Betamethasone Brand names include Betnelan, Betnesol, Betnovate, Bextasol, Diprosone, Vista-Methasone. Combined preparation brand names: Betnesol N, Betnovate C, Diprosalic and Fusibet.

2
The first step

Taking the first step in tackling any problem is probably the most difficult decision for most people. For the asthmatic who faces a bewildering array of 'patent medicines' on the shelf of the chemist, the health store, and now the super and hyper-market shelf, as well as numerous 'authorities' with conflicting ideas as to the management of asthma, it is doubly difficult. How long do you take a selected treatment before expecting results? Who should you consult for advice? It is hoped that these and many more questions will be answered before you reach the end of this book.

The very first step in clinical practice is to identify the problem, and it is no different in this instance. Only by an awareness of the causative factors, the aggravating factors, by an assessment of your general health, and by questioning whether your mental – emotional – and physical levels are in the best shape possible can you make a start. The best way is to prepare a list of questions and answer each question as honestly as you can. At the end of it you will be surprised to see that the problem areas are often quite clearly defined. Remember, every one of us is different, and each of us needs to amend and strengthen different areas in order to achieve health. Your best chances of success lie in a systematic approach that will eventually enable you to decide what adjustments need to be made in your life, plus what (if any) medicines or supplements may help your condition, and to come to a general awareness of yourself in relation to your asthma.

Too many sufferers in the past have not achieved the benefit they might have from alternative medicine for a number of reasons. Some have just tried at random one or two herbal medicines, some have tried taking vitamin supplements at random, when questioned as to why they tried them vaguely remembered 'reading it somewhere'!

Your health, and the control of your asthma, is far too important to just experiment with. Don't try only that which appeals to you – prepare a plan of action and then follow it for a set period of time. At the end of that period, if the improvement gained is worthwhile, then persist with your plan to see how much further you can improve.

The following headings are not meant as a complete questionnaire: they are a guide only. The questions are basic ones and it is hoped that you will find more of your own to add. Answer these questions and you will be taking the first step toward a new level of health.

What is health?

The state of health implies more than the freedom from disease. Good health may be defined as the attainment and maintenance of the highest state of mental and bodily vigour of which any given individual is capable.

Each of us is different, and whilst some have the potential to achieve glowing health and energy, others may have to be content with a lower plane of health. It is important that each person recognizes his or her own capabilities and achieves the maximum within that. An awareness of inherent weaknesses which may reduce capabilities in some spheres on either physical or mental levels should be recognized and allowed for. Having said that, it must not be used as an excuse for not trying, because unless you try, you will never know your true capabilities or the level of health that you should be enjoying.

Asthma and food

Many people eat for comfort, and the asthmatic is no exception. This applies especially to children. I cannot count the number of times that I have heard a mother confess that she has regularly given in to the demands of her asthmatic child for favourite foods such as sweets, chips, hamburgers, and Coke. It is a mistaken act of love and compassion toward a child who, by reason of the

asthma, cannot enjoy a 'normal' life. It allows an undermining of essential health by bad diet, which in turn may
cause a worsening of the asthma.

Many adult asthmatics will consume quantities of food
or alcohol that they know by experience aggravates their
condition. They eat to relieve a condition often nearing
depression, or is it apathy? Have they allowed their
general health to be undermined so much that they cannot
see a glimmer of light at the end of the tunnel? For many
with allergic asthma, the type of food they eat could be
vital to the control of their asthma, whilst the intrinsic
asthma sufferer needs to keep a healthy body in order to
ward off infection and reduce reaction to stress. Both
types of asthma can be helped with the correct foods, plus
vitamin supplements if needed, and herbal or homoeopathic medicines.

There are also a number of foods containing particular
preservatives or colourings which will produce an allergic
reaction in some people. This reaction can take place on
the skin, or more dangerously, it can affect the respiratory
system.

- **Question.** Am I aware of the foods that I should avoid
  in order to prevent an aggravation to my asthma?
- **Question.** Do I take particular care in choosing those
  foods that will give me all the necessary nutrients,
  minerals and vitamins for a healthy body?
- **Question.** Do I allow my child to dictate what food he
  or she will eat? Or do I follow a reasonable compromise,
  knowing that certain foods must be avoided, and look
  for acceptable alternatives?
- **Question.** Have I taken an allergy test to ascertain the
  foods that I may be allergic to?
- **Question.** Having discovered the allergic foods, do I
  avoid them?
- **Question.** Am I overweight? Could this be aggravating
  my asthma?

Asthma and work

Many asthmatics seem totally unaware of the possibility
that their working environment could be a cause in itself

for lost working hours due to asthma. Most people work under some form of stress, and it is important for all forms of asthma that you learn to cope with stress by replacing it with a relaxed and confident approach. Many people hate the work they do, and yet circumstances or cowardice often prevent them making that vital decision to seek a job in which they are happy, and which also suits their asthma. For instance, some asthmatics have a permanent cough from working in an environment in which they are constantly breathing in other people's cigarette smoke, or where the atmosphere is dry from an air-conditioning plant. Some asthmatics work in industry in atmospheres of dust or fumes, which in some cases have actually caused their condition. Some allergic asthma sufferers work on the land or in the parks among the pollens and grasses that they should be avoiding at all costs.

- **Question.** Does my work produce stress?
- **Question.** Does my workplace produce an atmosphere that I find difficult to breathe?
- **Question.** Am I an indoor or outdoor person: does my asthma improve dramatically in or out of doors?
- **Question.** When I return home from work am I relaxed and at ease?
- **Question.** Am I doing the kind of work that I enjoy and from which I get satisfaction?
- **Question.** Is my work within reasonable travelling distance of home?
- **Question.** Does my journey to work cause me stress?
- **Question.** Have I noticed if my asthma is better when I am at work or at home?

Asthma and school

For the child who suffers from asthma, school can be a source of dread or delight. It is good for the child, both emotionally and mentally, that it takes its place with other children in preparing for life. The school period, however, can be a nightmare for some, because stronger, less sensitive children will often 'pick on' the weaker ones, or those that are apart from the pack by reason of some abnormality. Some asthmatic children will use their asthma as an excuse to avoid certain lessons they dislike, or homework may be missed because they 'don't feel like it'. We would all like a reasonable excuse sometimes to get out of doing something we don't like, so who can blame a child who perhaps labours daily under a burden of breathing that prevents participation in normal activities? Some intrinsic asthma is definitely induced by physical activity and a number of children should be excused P.E.; for others who are not affected by physical activity the gymnasium nevertheless becomes a place of aggravation, due mainly to dust-coated floors and coconut matting, both of which give off clouds of particles kicked up by running feet.

During the school day most children are out of their parents' control: few come home to lunch. School lunches vary enormously from school to school; some provide an excellent variety of food whilst others exist on 'burgers and chips' type lunches. Children have been known to spend their lunch money regularly on crisps and sweets – to the asthmatic this could be disastrous and the cause of regular aggravation to the asthma.

- **Question.** Do I ensure to the best of my ability that my child is fully aware of the dangers of certain foods and will avoid them?
- **Question.** Have I as a parent ensured that the teachers and headmaster of the school are aware of the do's and don'ts necessary to prevent an asthma attack in my child?
- **Question.** Have I ensured that my child's teacher knows when during an asthma attack to call for professional help?
- **Question.** Do I regularly check that my child carries necessary medication to school daily in case of an attack?
- **Question.** Am I sensitive enough to my child's mental/ emotional well-being?
- **Question.** Do I encourage enough the effort to keep up with homework and school attendance within the reasonable capability of the asthmatic child?

- **Question.** Am I aware of the particular stress factors that aggravate my child's asthma?
- **Question.** Have I ensured that my child's friends are sympathetic to the asthma condition, and will quietly avoid the situations that may cause an attack?

Asthma and home

The living environment for an asthmatic is very important in many different ways. From the simple allergy point of view, the rooms in which the asthmatic spends most time – usually the living room and the bedroom – should be as dust-free as possible. Wall to wall carpeting can be particularly hazardous, as it traps dust which is released on vacuuming or with heavy pedestrian traffic. Heavy thick curtains hold dust and, during the winter, can release clouds of dust when opened or closed. The bedroom is important. Blankets of wool can release many small fibres undetected by the average person, but which to the asthmatic can mean a very uncomfortable night. Pillows can be stuffed with feathers which can cause a chronic allergic reaction. Pets should be chosen with care or not at all. Dogs, cats, and caged birds in the house can produce the necessary allergens to guarantee recurring asthma attacks in the susceptible asthmatic. Horses, rabbits and long-haired guinea pigs can also aggravate asthma.

Extrinsic asthmatics who live in or on the edge of the countryside find the summer a source of serious problems. Open windows allow in sprays from farms, pollens from trees and flowers whilst houseplants can produce a reaction in asthma both from their pollen and from the spores of mould produced in their soil.

- **Question.** Have I looked seriously at my home as a possible source of aggravation?
- **Question.** Do I make sure that my child has stuffed toys that are free from dust and fibre?
- **Question.** In the summer months do I take particular care to ensure the windows are kept shut?
- **Question.** Have I installed an ionizer?
- **Question.** Have I ensured that house pets are of the short-haired variety?

- **Question.** Have I educated my asthmatic child enough in what animals they must avoid cuddling or stroking?
- **Question.** Are my clothes chosen with enough care to give me maximum protection from fibres and hair?
- **Question.** If my asthma is bronchitic do I keep my house warm and aired properly to avoid sudden changes in temperature?
- **Question.** Do I monitor carefully enough the hours my child spends in front of the television set, and the correct balance of fresh air activity necessary for an asthmatic?
- **Question.** Could my houseplants be a source of aggravation to my asthma?

Asthma and holidays

The correct location of the holiday venue for an asthmatic can be very important.

The extrinsic asthmatic should choose a time and location which will be relatively free of the allergens which trigger an attack. As most airborne allergens are related to pollens or seed dust it will be obvious that the countryside in the early and midsummer months will produce an atmosphere laden with aggravating factors to the condition. The seaside, on the other hand, with its sea breezes and ozone, often brings great relief to the sufferer. Mountains also offer a reasonable atmosphere, provided they are not heavily wooded with fast-growing fir trees – this environment often creates an aggravation and so should be avoided. Swimming in the sea also provides bracing exercise, as will mountain walking if the air is clear and crisp.

Similar venues will also benefit the intrinsic asthmatic. The consideration in this case should be to avoid too strenuous a terrain which will overtax the strength and cause breathlessness.

The journey to the holiday should also be considered, for the allergic sufferer a long car journey through heavily pollenated countryside will produce symptoms, especially if the day is hot and the fan of the car is sucking in the allergen-laden air. Likewise, if travelling by aeroplane, seating in the non-smoking area should be arranged well in advance with the airline, and they should also be alerted to the fact that you do suffer with asthma. Very long flying times should be avoided if possible by planning several shorter flights, even if this means detouring from the direct route.

The intrinsic sufferer should avoid carrying heavy suitcases through miles of airport corridors. Most airports provide an electric cart with driver to transport both you and your luggage to the embarkation area. The airline will also arrange that you board the plane before or after the main crush of passengers embark. A little thoughtful forward planning can ensure a comfortable and stress-free flight.

- **Question.** Do I plan my holidays with enough care?
- **Question.** Have I isolated those locations which aggravate my asthma and do I avoid them?
- **Question.** Do I take into consideration when planning my holiday the correct time of the year which gives me the greatest freedom from asthma?
- **Question.** Do I ensure that the method of travel I have chosen is best suited to my asthma?
- **Question.** Do I ensure that I take enough medication with me for the duration of my holiday or, if travelling abroad, that the country to which I am travelling will have my medication available?
- **Question.** Do I ensure that I take out the correct medical insurance in case of emergency hospitalization abroad?

Asthma and pregnancy

As stated earlier, the chances of a baby being born with asthma are significantly increased if one parent is asthmatic, but the incidence of asthma developing in the child is dramatically increased if both parents suffer. The baby will be born with a far greater chance of overcoming the asthma tendency if the mother-to-be takes firm steps to improve her own health at the commencement of the pregnancy. She should also inform her obstetrician that she suffers from asthma. This will ensure that the correct drugs, and if necessary the correct type of anaesthetic, will be administered.

Some women actually feel much relief from their asthma during the pregnancy, due in some measure to the increase in certain hormones. Some women unfortunately find that their asthma worsens during pregnancy, or that they suffer other distressing conditions as well. One of the most common conditions to accompany pregnancy is heartburn; generally this is due to the uterus enlarging and putting pressure on the stomach, which in turn causes a backward flow of gastric juices. It is important to remember that some prescribed drugs used for the control of asthma may aggravate this heartburn. As this condition is mostly worse at night, the easiest method of alleviating it without the use of medicines is to raise the foot of the bed approximately six inches. In some women the increase of certain hormones during pregnancy can cause a form of chronic nasal congestion. The asthmatic should ask advice from the chemist before buying a decongestant over the counter, as some can cause aggravation to the asthma. A simple and harmless remedy for this condition is sniffing warm salt water.

Cigarette smoking should be avoided by all asthmatics, but most particularly by pregnant women. General health should be considered, because the health of the mother may reflect on the baby. The correct food and drink should be taken throughout the pregnancy – this means putting aside the fattening foods, reducing drastically the amount of tea and coffee that is drunk daily, and instead ensuring that you take plenty of fresh foods, salads, fruit, fruit drinks and mineral water daily, plus a good vitamin and mineral supplement. More information can be found regarding vitamins and minerals later in this book.

Regular daily exercise, both indoors and out must be taken; the amount, of course, will vary as the pregnancy progresses. Stress should be reduced as far as possible to the minimum and a little time set aside daily for relaxation, both mental and physical. Good quality sleep will round off for you a basic health programme which is essential throughout the pregnancy.

- **Question.** Am I taking enough care with my diet?
- **Question.** Do I ensure a regular daily exercise routine?

- **Question.** Have I stopped smoking?
- **Question.** Am I creating a relaxed and happy atmosphere around me each day?
- **Question.** Do I put aside a daily period for rest and relaxation?
- **Question.** Have I discussed my asthma and any asthma drugs that I may be taking in relation to my pregnancy with my doctor?
- **Question.** Have I ensured that the hospital are aware of my asthma?
- **Question.** Am I taking the correct vitamin/mineral supplement through my pregnancy?

Asthma and the elderly

It is generally recognized by medical authorities that we become more susceptible to illness and infection as we grow older, and so it becomes very important to try and maintain the best state of health possible. Not only will this enable you to enjoy life more, but it will also afford you a certain amount of protection against recurring infections.

Many older people suffer intrinsic asthma that has developed later in life, and is more common in women who have a history of wheezing and bronchitis. The older asthmatic will find that viral infections such as the common cold and flu can lead to a period of asthma, often several weeks after the infection, and so it makes sense to protect against these infections by keeping warm indoors during cold winter, well wrapped up against the winter weather if going out, and to ensure that a regular dietary pattern is followed: this means that at least one hot, nutritious meal a day is eaten. Extremes of temperature should be avoided, and heavy tobacco smoking should be stopped.

Many older people find that their income from pension funds and State pensions are often not enough to pay the many bills that periodically arrive on their doorstep, and they subsequently cut down on what they consider to be 'non-essentials'. Unfortunately this often means reducing their heating and food spending, which in turn gradually undermines their health, so that with the onset of the wet, damp and cold weather each winter they gradually slip lower in health. They are unaware of this at first, often only feeling a little more tired than usual, and feeling the cold a little more. It is at this stage they are most likely to catch a cold or flu which can then lead to bronchitis or pneumonia. Once this settles on the chest the asthma begins to worsen, and it is often a long, slow climb back to health. The more frequently this happens, the weaker the chest becomes, and the more frequent the asthma attacks become. Often an older person with such a history will have a permanent 'wheeze'.

Some older people also develop diabetes, and in some cases this will lead to an asthma condition developing.

There is another form of asthma, called *cardiac asthma*, to which older people can be prone. The symptoms are sudden attacks of shortness of breath while the person is resting. This is a very serious symptom, and could be due to severe heart failure. If your symptoms are similar, immediate medical help should be sought.

Some people have an allergy to aspirin or aspirin-based medicines – if you have such an allergy and are also an asthmatic you must be careful not only to avoid aspirin, but also some non-steroidal anti-inflammatory drugs. It is simple to ask your doctor not to prescribe these, but the danger lies in buying medicines over the counter which often contain *acetylsalicylic acid*: this is aspirin, which can be found in many common cold remedies. You should always read the label carefully before buying such medicines.

Stress is another cause of asthma; in older people stress is often caused by worrying about such things as their health, or money problems, or everyday problems like filling in official forms correctly. Even dealing with local authorities, the maintenance of the elderly person's home, or loneliness can cause a form of stress.

- **Question.** Do I ensure that I protect myself in the winter by wearing warm clothing?
- **Question.** Do I pay enough attention to eating at least one warm nutritious meal daily during the winter months?

- **Question.** Do I monitor carefully enough the amount of cigarettes or tobacco I smoke daily?
- **Question.** Do I ensure that I am not under stress by asking someone to help if I am in need of assistance of any kind?
- **Question.** Do I try and lead a full life free of loneliness by, for example, joining associations that will lead to friendships?
- **Question.** Do I take enough regular exercise?
- **Question.** Do I give priority to buying the correct foods?
- **Question.** Do I find that my money does not cover all the bills and food and heating?
- **Question.** Am I willing to discuss any financial problem with the Social Services?
- **Question.** If I am allergic to aspirin, do I check carefully the ingredients of all medicines before I buy them?

3
The next step

If you have selected the questions that were relevant to you and answered them, you should now have before you a list of those areas that you have neglected or not thought of before as being important. The following chapters outline the different therapies and dietary suggestions that will help you to adjust positively those areas of your physical and mental self and help toward an improvement of the quality of your life.

The power of positive thinking

'Positively' is an interesting word, it suggests a definite approach, a determination to try, a 'putting aside' of the apathy that encroaches on our lives without us being aware of it.

Many people who have suffered asthma for years adopt a way of life, sometimes of necessity, that allows the least aggravation to their symptoms. Of course this is essential in some cases, but the purpose of this chapter is to look at the attitude of mind that accompanies that decision. For instance, do you restrict yourself with determination or with resignation from doing things that may aggravate your asthma?

The fact that you have progressed so far into the pages of this book implies that you are interested in trying to help yourself. That is the first step. The next step is to look at your list of questions and start at the first negative answer.

For example, let us suppose that you are male, approximately 40 years of age, married with 3 children. Your first negative answer concerns your attitude to work. You find it difficult, a 'drag' to say the least. Ask yourself 'why?'.

Did you find your work interesting and exciting when you first started? If the answer is 'yes', why do you now find it 'a drag'? Is it the environment? Could it be that you have been passed over for promotion in favour of somebody that you don't particularly like? Do you feel capable of better things? Maybe you have lost sight of the reason that you work in the first place.

This is the difficult point in the exercise; you must now try and answer the question you have posed.

Let us take the first possibility, that you have been passed over for promotion. You need to examine the reasons without emotion, as if someone else were reading the question; then you may find the reasons begin to emerge. You may need to admit that the person promoted in your place was better qualified than you, and that if you were the boss your choice would probably be the same. Or could it be that despite your qualifications for the position, your attitude to your work ('a drag') had been noticed by those above you? In this case the reason for losing the post would lie directly with you, and your own 'negative vibrations'.

To lose sight of the reason for doing something important in life such as working is really quite serious. It implies that you may have reached the 'zombie' stage. You must look closely into your attitude in order to fully understand where you may have gone wrong.

Most of us work to earn money – that is the basic reason that everyone must equate with. We in turn earn the money to pay for those things in life such as rent or mortgage, food, clothes, education, which we in the western world consider necessities. In achieving this, a certain amount of pleasure should be gained simply because you are supplying your basic needs and, if you have one, also supporting a family. As your abilities and income increase, so will the ability to buy the extras: holidays, restaurant meals, theatre or cinema visits, or just saving a nest egg. These are the simple reasons for which we work.

This form of self-analysis can be disturbing, for often we have lost the ability to 'enjoy' without realizing it, and discover through self-analysis that we live almost in a state of depression.

What can I do? The power of positive thinking

Positive thinking produces a power in itself, a power which in some subtle way is felt by others around. You must have met the person who, when they enter a room, makes heads turn not because they dress in expensive or outlandish clothes, but because they exude a certain 'power'. Remember, when you make the decision to alter your habits or lifestyle you are practising positive thought and some of that 'power' begins to work right away in you.

I am not suggesting that you will achieve total health just by positive thinking, but positive thinking does produce positive action, and that is precisely what this book is about. Thought is a living thing; it has a vibration and travels to where it is directed. Imagine a thought as a pebble which is dropped into the middle of a perfectly still pond. From it, ripples spread out in increasingly wider circles until they reach the edge of the pond. If you watch carefully those ripples then begin to return to the middle from where they first came.

Picture your thoughts going out like a ripple from your mind and eventually coming back to you. Then realize that if they were negative thoughts of dislike or resentment at somebody, they have gone out like ripples and are returning to bombard you, and so you become the centre of your own negative thoughts!

Imagine your thoughts are positive, filled with care and concern for those around you, that you are happy and contented in all that you do. Those thought waves are continually coming back at you and bathing you continuously in happy vibrations. From this you will understand why some people are always unhapppy, and some always happy even though they don't appear to have anything to be happy about.

The power of positive thought is more than just a catch-phrase – it can be the secret to success and happiness in life, just as negative thoughts can bring depression and despair.

How can I begin?

Start by remembering that you are a free person and, if employed, that you contracted your particular skills of your own free will, to a person or company in return for an agreed sum of money per year. Whether employed or self-employed, remember that your work should take only a certain amount of your time per day: before work and after work, your time is yours.

Acknowledge that the way in which you spend that time often colours your entire thinking.

For instance, many people rise from bed in the morning with just enough time to wash, dress, perhaps eat a little breakfast, and then travel to work. By the time they reach work they have had little time to adjust from bed, and so their work commences, as far as they are concerned, almost from the moment they rise. They perform their work, take a period for lunch and eventually arrive home.

At home a routine often takes place which has become a habit, perhaps a period in front of the television set of just 'letting go', is then followed by preparing and eating the evening meal. Following a meal, most of us experience a feeling of lethargy as our bodies begin the digestive processes. We then relax in a chair, which is often placed conveniently near a television set. Our mind focuses in a lethargic way on whatever particular programme happens to be showing, or by habit we know what is showing, and settle down comfortably to watch a programme which we will often deny to our work colleagues that we do watch. Several hours in front of the television set, our evening meal digested, leads conveniently to the appropriate time to retire to bed.

Can you wonder that this person often feels a great deal of suppressed anger or frustration with life? As far as they are concerned, life has become meaningless.

Can you see a familiar pattern developing? Has your world become small and uninteresting? If so, there are some positive changes in your attitude and thinking needed.

You have already started your plan of action by writing down those changes you have decided are needed in your life. This will of course vary from individual to individual:

some will find only minor changes are needed to bring improvement to their asthma and a sparkle to their smile, while others may decide that major changes are needed, and these of course can take time. If you always keep a mental picture of what you wish to achieve, however, time will pass more quickly than you think.

To return to your list, I would suggest that you make the three following headings on a separate sheet of paper:

Physical – Mental – Emotional

Then look at each answer in turn and if something needs to be improved in your life, enter it under the appropriate heading. This will bring order into what otherwise could look a bewildering heap of answers. Do you remember first attempting a jigsaw puzzle? You probably sorted through all the pieces looking for a particular one, only it often took a long time. To make things easy you sorted the pieces of the jigsaw into different piles before attempting the puzzle, and this made it much easier to complete the picture. In the same manner, by sorting your problems into different piles they will assume their correct proportions, and be that much easier to sort out.

Remember!

- It is always better to attempt one change at a time, so that you do not overstrain either your energies or your abilities.

- Having started, see it through, as determination itself can be a positive force.

- By following these two simple rules you will guarantee succes in whatever you wish to achieve.

The three headings

Physical   Under this heading could be grouped changes that are needed in the home, or at work and changes in your physical approach to life such as exercise, recreation, and holidays. Also under this heading would come the type of therapy you may choose to manage your asthma, as well as diet changes and the addition of supplements such as vitamins and minerals if indicated. Giving up smoking will also come under this heading, and for the elderly it could mean arranging the heavy tasks in a different way, and looking at ways of increasing the enjoyment of life.

Mental For some this is not an easy area to define: what is the difference between mental and emotional?

Your mental approach is the way in which you tackle life. For instance, do you decide to do something and then do it? Or do you hesitate, anxious in case you may fail or be doing the wrong thing?

Your emotional reaction is the feeling of hurt if a friend or colleague says something against you.

Your mental attitude is applied to your work, to your superiors and inferiors. Do you resent taking orders? Do you try and do as little work as possible for the maximum money you can get?

Do you allow your asthma to become an excuse to avoid social engagements with friends or acquaintances? Do you get up each morning dreading the day ahead? Attitudes such as unnecessary irritability, ingratitude, being too demanding, and peevishness would classify in this heading also.

Emotional Negative feelings come under this heading, such as hate, jealousy, guilt and anger. Fear is an emotion, as are anxiety and temper. Depression can be caused by a lack of emotion; your attitude to a loved one, if negative, would also come under this heading.

Be careful not to allow emotional feelings to enter your work time, as they will invariably end up as negative feelings.

You should now have before you the three categories containing the things in your life which need changing. You should assemble them in neat lists and start at the beginning of each list, and only move on to the next weakness when you are satisfied that you have corrected the one you are working on.

4
Mental relaxation and stress control

Our mind plays a vital role in our health. Looking at some of the sayings that have developed over the years, such as 'you make me sick', 'you get on my nerves', etc. is a good illustration of the effect that we allow other people to have on our physical health. If you study a healthy person, not only do they appear to be physically fit but they also have a positive state of mind. They are enthusiastic toward life, happy in any environment, interested in their work, and generally succeed in all they attempt. On the other hand the person who has not enjoyed good health often has a negative approach to life: they are not interested in sports or hobbies, find socializing an effort, and generally become withdrawn and introvert. This raises an interesting question: did their negative state of mind contribute to their illness, or did the illness cause the negative state of mind?

Is the saying 'we are what we think' true? If so, what part does stress play in our thinking?

What is stress?

It is important to first define and recognize stress in order to treat it, and so we ask 'what is stress?'.

Stress is the individual's reaction to a particular environment or situation in which they are not happy, and which they think they have little power to change. Stress is the inability to direct the working of the mind away from negative thought, or to control pent-up anger or frustration.

The cause of stress varies considerably from person to person, and the interesting fact is that what constitutes stress for one person does not necessarily affect another.

What causes stress?

There are two main categories of stress. The first is direct stress – this is the kind of everyday stress which is easily recognizable; the second is subliminal stress, the kind which we are often unaware of until it begins affecting us.

Direct stress

A friend or a loved one can upset us with a cross word and change our entire day, making us feel low or angry and unwanted. Our thoughts and emotions then become our enemy by being negative. A difficult journey to work can often result in a bad mood, causing us when we arrive to be short-tempered, and this in turn will often spark a similar response from those around us. In this way we become producers of our own stress which continues to feed on itself, like the ripples of a pond as mentioned in the previous chapter.

In the west today, we have become success-orientated, and much of our life is taken up with achieving either rank or status in order to impress others, in the so-called 'rat race' which is responsible for producing both mental and physical stress.

Subliminal stress

This comes in a number of different forms, such as the continuing news reports of violence and death, or of nations suffering deprivation from major catastrophes and war, that are constantly fed into our subconscious minds. Some people have bad neighbours, for example, or suffer stressful relationships at home with close family. These factors subconsciously influence the way we feel, and lead to subliminal stress.

Having studied the behavioural patterns of people over a number of years, I have concluded there must be a common denominator to subliminal stress. One predominant factor appears to be an element of fear which is inherent in each of us to some degree. We are born *without* fear on the physical plane, but we have fear instilled into us during the growing years to preserve us from harm. For instance, we are taught to fear and respect fire as it has the potential to hurt or kill. Unwittingly, during our formative years we develop a fear of the dark as we are regaled with stories of ghosts and bogey men. As we develop and grow we are encouraged by our parents to strive and better ourselves; in some cases this is beyond the capability of the child and can produce stress. The tendency over the past several decades to build houses in closer proximity to each other has meant living in larger communities; we also travel and work in more crowded conditions. All of this produces less and less privacy: our 'own space' becomes smaller and this produces a subliminal atmosphere of tension. In this increasing tension, where each of us feels under microscopic scrutiny, the individual needs to be seen to succeed. This in turn can produce an underlying fear of 'not succeeding', or a 'fear of failure' which is common to each of us in varying degrees. You can observe this in a number of subtle ways. For instance, some people do not like attending social occasions, and when questioned as to why, they will often admit to 'feeling out of place'. In other words 'not easy in company', they worry about the impression that others may have of them, or that they will be talked about behind their back. This fear of not being liked causes them to avoid these situations which are likely to bring them into confrontation with their fear.

There are others who have not succeeded in their professional life as they would have wished, often blaming their failure for promotion on others who have 'stepped over them'. This leads to bottled-up resentment which can be a major cause of stress. If you question them closely you will often find that there have been numerous occasions in the past when they should have exerted authority and spoken out or reprimanded a colleague, but failed to do so for fear of failure or fear of what others would think of them.

And so fear becomes a part of our programmed response to situations and people, and this produces subliminal stress. Fortunately, the majority of adults have managed to rationalize their childhood fears and can see them in proper perspective, but the more subtle fears are not so easy to rationalize and they continue to influence our lives and sometimes our health in a negative way.

This causes us to feel 'uptight' within ourselves, and is often revealed in our body language. Body language is the tendency we have to form physical habit patterns around our stress; for instance, you can often spot an asthmatic by their habit of breathing in short bursts with their shoulders hunched. This is a reflection of the continuing anxiety syndrome which is experienced during an attack and which the subconscious mind has allowed to develop into a physical habit.

The importance of our body language

Try looking at people around you and observe their 'body language'. The slope of the shoulders, a bent or straight back, the line of a mouth, as well as the lines around the eyes and on the forehead can reveal a person's inner character in moments.

Check your own body language in the first shop window or mirror that you pass. What does it say to you?

Do you read positive signs such as tranquillity, kindness and consideration? Do the lines around your eyes and mouth turn up in a happy way or down in a frown? Do you stand easy, with shoulders straight and head high, or does the slump of your shoulders reveal the weight of our inner troubles?

Ask yourself: are you a prime candidate for stress? Have you lost the ability to relax and enjoy life?

Anticipation

Another form of subliminal stress is the way in which we actually build stress before it arrives: this is called anticipation. How often have you experienced a restless night because you were worrying about something that was going to happen the next day? (A dentist's appointment? An interview with the boss? A driving test?) By the time the appointment arrives you have worked yourself into a 'state of nerves'.

For the asthmatic this can lead to a worsening of the asthma, because the stress causes an increasing tightness of the chest which promotes further anxiety, and eventually an asthma attack will develop.

Stress has been acknowledged as one of the foremost

dangers to health in the modern world, and it can be a killer! Many diseases in the present era are either caused or aggravated by stress, and among them is asthma. Experts have acknowledged that the incidence of asthma is definitely increasing, and so far they have not discovered the reason. Without doubt environmental pollution, and perhaps diet, play a part, but the largest factor in my opinion is stress.

Most people are unaware of the tangle of stress that surrounds them but they are still affected by it. It is hoped that the reader will recognize some of their own stress factors in this chapter and be able to deal effectively with them using some of the suggestions outlined here.

Controlling asthma through the mind

Stress control should form a part of your self-help programme, for by building a calm and relaxed mental attitude in life, you will help your asthma and benefit as an individual.

People who feel relaxed and calm within themselves act as a magnet to those around them. They are sought after for their opinion, succeed more easily in business, and generate a sense of harmony and well-being wherever they go.

It is important to understand that our reaction to stress takes place in our mind before it manifests in a physical form, i.e. in such diseases as asthma.

We have learnt that our reactions are influenced in some measure by the pre-conditioning of the conscious and subconscious which commenced in childhood. This in turn has led to fears and inhibitions which conditions our responses, and in some situations cause us to feel a great deal of unnecessary stress and anxiety through feelings of fear or inadequacy.

We have come to understand that many of our conditioned responses are in fact habits that we have acquired unconsciously. Some of these habits are positive, but some are negative. Stress control offers a way of eliminating these negative responses and replacing them with positive vibrations.

What is the mind?

The mind is a complex mechanism, but it can be simplified by separating it into two sections which are called the *conscious* and *subconscious*.

To control the mind and therefore our conscious and subconscious self is one of the greatest achievements that we can attain: through it we can overcome fears and inhibitions and, by positive thought, help to produce a state of physical health.

The conscious mind

Your conscious mind is at this moment reading the words on this page, and as you read you are accepting or rejecting the ideas and statements before you. The information which is accepted is then passed to the subconscious mind where it is stored for future reference. The conscious mind will accept or reject an idea by comparing it with already stored reference memories, these in turn have been acquired by our 'acceptance or rejection' ability. The conscious mind is the level of your brain which is constantly monitoring every message that it receives from your sensory organs, the eyes, ears, nose, and the touch and taste senses. According to its pre-programming it acts on this continuous flow of information, but if we are tired, or under stress, our ability to deal with this constant stream of information is weakened, and we become irritable and sometimes irrational. One of the symptoms of the conscious mind under stress is its inability to concentrate. It has a tendency to jump from subject to subject, it feeds negative thoughts to the subconscious, and eventually loses its ability to switch off at sleep periods.

The mind then begins to file anxiety reactions against situations that before were tranquil; its memory recall becomes weakened and we experience periods of forgetfulness. This means that we lose the ability to bring to the surface facts which we need from the filing systems below and we become 'absentminded'.

Most of us have minds that jump about from subject to subject, and often we are unable to follow a continuous train of thought without great difficulty; this becomes noticeably worse when we are under stress.

We find that when trying to relax, our thoughts will run off on a tangent causing us to dwell on memories, and soon we are experiencing past tensions as well as present ones. This is undesirable, as it prevents us from letting go of the tensions and giving our mind the essential rest period it must have in a similar way to the physical body.

The procedure needed to control these random wanderings of the thought processes is in essence quite simple, and yet to many it presents one of the most difficult exercises.

The subconscious mind

This is an area of the brain which has caused controversy among experts for centuries. Our subconscious reaction to our environment and situations is known to be the cause of stress as well as emotional upset, and yet it remains a mystery.

To understand a little of the subconscious we need to understand that it does not have the discriminating ability of the conscious mind, it simply acts as a storehouse for all the information which is passed to it from the conscious mind. Within it are stored our memories and impressions of life. Painful memories are locked away down here, as well as the sensory impressions and associations both seen, heard, felt, smelled or tasted.

Habit patterns are formed in the subsconscious by the simple process of repetition. For instance each time the subconscious receives an impression it files it away, and the more frequently it receives the same impression, the higher up the scale of importance it is placed and the more readily it responds to the stimulus.

Let us say for simplicity that it contains two sections which are labelled 'nice' and 'nasty'. If you eat something which disagrees with your digestion or the taste does not suit your palate, it will be placed in the section labelled 'nasty'. This will ensure that you do not repeat the experience. Likewise, a similar category is built up in the file marked 'nice', but unlike the 'nasty' file, the subconscious encourages you to repeat the 'nice' experiences. Unfortunately because of its inability to discriminate it will often file under 'nice' things which are not good for you, such as certain foods, cigarettes, alcohol, etc. Many of these 'habits' we have built slowly without realizing their importance until they begin to affect us adversely. A good example of this is cigarette smoking. Many people who smoke desperately want to stop, but the subconscious mind continues to produce the command for a cigarette whenever a stimulus it recognizes appears. This can be a particular time of day, for instance after food, or during a telephone conversation. It is also more noticeable during periods when stress is increased.

Responses such as this can be changed from the 'nice' category to the 'nasty' by undergoing hypnosis, or by establishing a new 'positive' habit in place of the 'negative' one.

This re-categorizing of 'habit patterns' can be simply achieved by using mind control.

Achieving mind control

Mental relaxation

To commence mind training you need to achieve a state of mental relaxation, a state of mind in which mental activity is reduced to a minimum and then guided along a definite path of thought. To commence it is advisable to choose a quiet place, preferably somewhere you know you will not be interrupted.

Either recline comfortably on your back, or in an armchair, and ensure that any tight clothing has been loosened. Relax your body by closing your eyes, and imagine that your feet are growing heavy. As soon as you feel they are heavier, proceed in a similar manner to make the legs heavy. Then concentrate on your buttocks and low back, and eventually proceed to the shoulders, following down both arms to your fingertips trying to imagine they are too heavy to lift. Move up to the neck and back of your head letting go of all the tensions of the day.

Keep your eyes closed throughout this exercise to shut out anything visual that might distract your mental concentration. Then imagine your abdomen is relaxing. This is the area 'below the belt', which contains the *solar plexus*, otherwise known as the 'sun centre' of the body. This is the most important area to control because from here radiates all 'tension' or 'tranquillity'. It is a very important area in mind control, for by learning to relax this part of your body, with a little practice you will be able to produce almost instant feelings of physical and mental relaxation.

If you find physical relaxation difficult, it sometimes helps to lie on your back and place a small coin on the centre of your forehead. Close your eyes and concentrate on your breathing, and you should soon find the body is relaxing.

Breathing control

Both mental and physical relaxation are comparatively easy to achieve in a quiet and relaxed atmosphere, but stress often occurs when we do not have access to such places. It is therefore most important to learn to relax in the centre of the stress, and to do this one must have a trigger which produces an instant feeling of mental tranquillity. The most important thing in life to the asthmatic is breathing. Most people use only 50 to 60 per cent of their lung capacity, and the asthmatic often uses much less. For the asthmatic, breathing is the obvious trigger, because by linking a breathing technique to your mind control exercises you are building a 'habit pattern' in the subconscious mind which will have a 'double positive' effect. It works by association: as you have already learned, the subconscious has no reasoning power, but responds to triggers. If lunch is always served at 1pm, the mind begins to associate 1pm with food and you become hungry. In a similar way, if the mind associates mental relaxation with a special form of breathing, then whenever you switch to that form of breathing you will find the mind releases its stress.

To achieve this means daily training in both the breathing and mental exercises.

Breathing technique

This is based on a form of yoga breathing which is both deep and slow. You can breathe through your mouth or nose *and remember it is a slow breath in as well as out*. The control for the breathing is in the throat just behind the tongue; by narrowing this area a little you restrict the passage through which the air passes to the lungs. This creates an effect as if you were breathing through a straw, the air is compressed and rushes into the lungs with a greater velocity which causes them to fill from the bottom first, this is most beneficial to the asthmatic as it provides more oxygen with less effort.

When you have mastered the technique your breathing will have a new sound to it, rather like listening to someone who is deeply asleep. Also you will feel a cold sensation at the back of the tongue when breathing in, as if the air were rushing out.

This means that you can test your breathing technique in two ways, by sound and sensation. After one or two of these deep breaths it is quite normal to feel somewhat dizzy, this is a signal to stop for a while. The slight feeling of dizziness is caused by the increased amount of oxygen which the lungs are absorbing; the more you practise the less you will notice this symptom.

This deep breathing method fills the lungs completely and causes the expanded lungs to act like balloons, they fill the chest and without effort you will find that your spine adopts a more upright stance. This can be of special benefit to the asthmatic in overcoming a tendency to curvature of the spine which develops as a result of shallow breathing. The more upright stance which follows also allows the head to be held higher, which of course frees pressure on the windpipe and adds to the freedom of breathing.

- Never strain to breathe deeply; always breathe easily, without effort, and stop when you feel strain commencing.

Practising your breathing

An athlete trains to increase his lung capacity to provide more oxygen to cope with the demands he is about to make on his body. In a similar manner the asthmatic needs to train his lungs in order to increase their capacity and utilize every ounce of oxygen to compensate for a restricted lung capacity.

Breathing is one of the body's automatic functions, that means that it does not need a conscious command to breathe.

However, in this method of breathing control you are going to bring your breathing under your 'conscious' control for a time and reprogram the subconscious by introducing a positive habit in place of a negative one. The negative habit is that of laboured asthma breathing, the positive is a growing awareness and appreciation of each deep breath that you take. Try to become aware of its life-giving oxygen as it flows into your lungs bringing with it a sense of well-being at all times.

It is important to practise daily at a regular time that you know is always free. If you have difficulty finding such a time, inform those around you that it is important to your health programme that you have this period free. Hang a notice on your door to remind people that you do not wish to be disturbed; only in this way will you be able to really relax and concentrate.

It is also important to practise just before going to sleep. Not only is the body relaxing, but the subconscious is programmed for sleep, and so will be more receptive to relaxation. If you commence practising about five minutes before your normal sleep time you will find the body slips into deep sleep much more quickly, and the breathing throughout the night will be easier.

For those readers who snore, this method of breathing control will quickly overcome the tendency. A snore is simply the same type of deep breathing but with the throat narrowed at the wrong place.

Breathing awareness

During the day at intervals of approximately half an hour you should make yourself aware of your breathing for a few moments, and consciously take a few 'special deep breaths'.

When out walking you can practise 'rhythmic breathing' – this is a technique of bringing the breathing and the heart beat into harmony, it produces a feeling of relaxation and well-being within a few minutes. Begin by counting how many footsteps you take while taking one deep in-breath, then hold that in-breath for half the number of footsteps it took you to breathe in. The breath out should take the same number of footsteps it took to breathe in. Using this practice method you will soon find that you are able to walk much further, with greater ease of breathing, and with an upright body.

Another technique of bringing the heart beat into harmony with the breathing is performed while sitting and relaxing, perhaps whilst watching a television programme. Either place your hand over your heart so that you can feel it beating, or with the first two fingers of one hand feel your wrist pulse which is situated on the inside of the wrist in a direct line with the thumb. Commence taking a special deep breath while counting the number of heart beats it takes to completely fill your lungs, hold the breath for half that number, then breathe out while counting the same number as you took to breathe in.

With daily practice you will find that your lung capacity slowly increases and your body feels more relaxed. These are signs that you are making progress, you should continue the breathing and physical relaxation until you feel you have control. Then it will be time to move on to the next phase:

Mind control

This part of the exercise presents a greater challenge and is more difficult. Through the technique outlined you will be endeavouring to change those 'negative' habits into a 'positive' mental response.

Most of us have some ability to make mental pictures: for instance, when reading a novel we illustrate it by building a constantly changing picture in our minds. To test your ability for making mental pictures, close your eyes and see if you can imagine a pale blue Rolls Royce motor car with large pink spots all over it. Behind the wheel is a thin-faced man with beard, wearing a bright green top hat. If you managed to produce that picture for a short time in your mind, you should benefit from the following mind control exercises.

If you are one of the few people who cannot visualize mental pictures, there is a different mental exercise for you at the end of this chapter.

Any mind control programme that is to be followed regularly must be interesting to the individual. For this reason the following programme has several stages. Ideally, each one should be mastered before attempting the next; however, if you reach a stage and find the next is too difficult, it doesn't matter: providing you practise daily at one of the stages you will achieve your goal.

Stage one

Each of us has a favourite place which brings us a feeling of peace and tranquillity when we visit it. For some it is the sea, a walk on the shore, or a bracing walk along the cliffs. For others it is the countryside on a spring or summer day: fields, woodland, and solitude.

To commence stage one it is important to go through your physical relaxation programme accompanied by the special breathing. When the body is relaxed and you are breathing deeply without strain, quietly enter your mind and commence building a place of peace and tranquillity. It is important that you do not choose a favourite place and simply remember what it looks like, as this may lead to memories of past visits, and this in turn will allow the mind to start wandering. This is the very thing you are trying to overcome, and so your walk must be a new one, perhaps made up of little segments of favourite walks from the past, but the whole presenting a place that you have never been to before.

Then you must learn to place 'triggers'. These are parts of your walk which stand out a little more than the rest. At these points you stop and practise deeper relaxation, and in this way the conscious mind is gradually programmed to a state of progressive relaxation at each trigger.

Each of us will have different walks that are secret to us and tailored to fit our individual need.

The following exercise is simply an illustration to guide you and is not meant as part of the programme.

Try and quieten your mind as much as possible and imagine that you are standing in a field. There are hedgerows surrounding it on three sides; on the fourth side is a woodland with large mature trees spaced well apart. It is late spring, and the field which has never been ploughed or cut is full of wild flowers, herbs and grasses. You are sitting on the grass and feeling its cool touch on your hands; the smell of the grass mingles with the smell of the earth and wild flowers. The sky is blue with just little puffs of white cloud, the sun is warm on your skin, and you can hear the buzz of insects and the chirping of birds.

Still in your mind, lie on your back and close your eyes. Tune in to as many of the smells and sounds of the field as you can. Be aware of how your body feels lying on the grass. Then rise and wander around your field, look for clumps of flowers or herbs that you will recognize when you come again, look for bird nests in the hedge, or just sit very quietly letting go of the deep physical and mental tensions.

This completes stage one. During the exercise you have managed to make your mind work along a line of single thought controlled totally by yourself, and at the same time you have managed body control and taken over your breathing patterns. If you found your mental pictures kept fading, or they were not very clear, do not worry; simply continue your daily control exercises and you will find the pictures eventually become easier and easier to produce.

Stage two

When you find that you can mentally produce your favourite walk easily, the time has come to attempt stage two. This means expanding the walk and commencing to use the 'triggers'. We shall continue to illustrate with the fields and woodland.

The field lies before you, the day is bright and sunny, and the birds are singing. There is a patch of grass that is much shorter than the rest: here you sit and rest and let the tensions of the day slip away from your shoulders and neck. This is a trigger place, so take time to ensure you feel totally relaxed in the shoulders and neck.

Moving on, imagine a faint path across the field that leads to the woodland. As you walk, continue to build colour, sound and smell into your picture. As you approach the woodland notice each individual tree, the shape of it as well as the colour and shape of its leaves. You have now reached the woodland and you can see a path leading through it. The path is of beaten earth, and as you walk on it notice how different it feels from the grass of the field. Notice also the earthy smell of the woodland and how different that is from the smell of the field. The sound is different from the field's: in a woodland, sound echoes and is magnified. The breeze can no longer be felt on the skin; instead you can hear it brushing the leaves above you. A little way along the path, and to one side, lies a fallen tree trunk. This is a trigger point, and here you rest for a while sitting with your back resting against the fallen tree, and letting the deep muscles of your abdomen relax.

Continuing along the path, you eventually reach a stream. Grass grows along the water's edge, and across the stream is an old bridge. The stream is too wide to jump, although it is shallow and clean. Here you rest sitting by the water watching the play of sunlight flickering on its moving surface, seeing the reflection of the trees above and patches of blue sky. Then in your mind lie on the grass by the stream and look up through the trees to the sky, allow your eyes to close and listen to the sound of the stream as the water flows gently between its banks. This is a trigger point and you should now try and imagine that your body is a part of the stream and that you are floating with it, try and encourage all tension to float away from your body. Completing stage two you should have felt a greater degree of relaxation at each trigger point.

Stage three

To achieve stage one or two your body was relaxed either by lying or sitting before both breathing and mental techniques were practised. Stage three is an extension of the first two stages, and is the practice of visiting your walk for 5 or 10 seconds only at any time during the day. You would choose a time in which your concentration would not be required on the physical level. For instance when sitting at your desk, or washing up at the sink, simply close your eyes for a second or two and switch on your deep breathing, and visualize a small part of your walk. A further stage of advancement is achieved by switching on your breathing and with eyes open, bringing a faint picture of a part of your walk on to the 'screen' of your mind.

Eventually you will not need the mental pictures of your walk, as switching on the special breathing will produce the total feeling of relaxation and mental tranquillity instantly, wherever you are. When you attain this stage of advancement you should be using the technique in short bursts throughout your working day to maintain a perfectly relaxed aura. Should you experience the commencement of an asthma attack, there is every reason to hope that you will manage to control it with the techniques illustrated.

Mind control without visualization

For those who just cannot form mental pictures there are other methods of training the mind to work along a single line of thought. The same physical relaxation and special breathing techniques are used together with the following techniques to prevent the mind wandering.

Stage one

The counting method – this is a simple method, but it is effective. I often use it in the clinic to help induce hypnosis in subjects who cannot concentrate visually. Commence by relaxing the physical body, and then with eyes closed adjust your breathing to the yoga breathing technique, then commence counting from 300 backwards in twos to the rhythm of your breathing.

Example After you have slowly and deeply filled the lungs, say out loud 'three hundred', then slowly empty the lungs.

When the lungs are completely empty say quite slowly and out loud 'two hundred and ninety eight', then commence to slowly fill the lungs again. So you will be building a pattern of breathing and counting; in breath – 300 – out breath – 298 – in breath – 296 – out breath 294. This continues until you reach zero, by which time you should feel totally relaxed, and your mind has had a time of training along a line of single thought. Alternatively, you will have drifted into a relaxed mental state which no longer requires counting.

After some weeks of practice you will find that you no

longer need to count: your breathing rhythm will be sufficient to produce a relaxed state.

Stage two

A lighted candle can be placed at a convenient point to enable you to fix your eyes comfortably upon it whilst physically relaxing the body and commencing the special breathing. Eventually a deeper state of relaxation can be attained by closing the eyes and retaining the picture of the candle flame.

Practice time

It is suggested that you commence with ten- or fifteen-minute periods in the day, and five- to ten-minute periods before sleep. These can be slowly extended over a period of weeks to thirty-minute periods during the day and a fifteen-minute period before sleep.

Using the relaxation techniques

For an asthma attack

The moment you experience the first symptoms of an asthma attack you should stop what you are doing. Take a quick stock of yourself to check that you are as physically relaxed as possible. Commence slow, deep breathing, and tell yourself that your breathing is slowly getting easier and easier. If necessary, close your eyes and try to visualize yourself in some pleasant tranquil surroundings. To assist the breathing, with every in-breath, slowly expand the chest by pushing your arms with elbows bent, backwards as far as you can.

Asthma at night

Should you awaken at night with asthma symptoms, the first thing to remember is *don't panic*. It sometimes helps to stand by the bed and begin the slow breathing exercises. If you cannot stand, do try and relax arms, shoulders and chest when lying in bed. Make sure that your mouth is not covered by sheet or blanket. With every 'in' breath that you take, try and arch the low part of your back, as this assists the chest to expand and you will get more oxygen.

Asthma at school

At the first symptoms of asthma at school, keep calm. If you are in a classroom ask the teacher's permission to leave for a moment. Try and get to some fresh air, and begin practising yoga breathing, at the same time letting your shoulder and stomach muscles go limp. Always remain within easy reach of help should you need it.

Games where short bursts of energy are used such as sprinting, cycling, long jump, cricket and swimming are particularly good for asthmatics.

Advice for parents

Do ensure that your child's teacher is fully aware of the condition, and of your child's need to carry medication; also ensure that the teacher knows how the medication should be administered during an asthma attack.

Ensure that the teacher is aware that long distance running, as well as strenuous games such as tennis, hockey, and badminton, are likely to induce an attack, and that the chances of an attack are heightened if the air is cold or dry, or if your child is suffering from a cold. During an attack your child should be allowed to relax away from other children and must be supervised while taking asthma drugs.

If the symptoms do not subside within five minutes, or the child has blue lips, an ambulance should be called immediately.

If your child has exercise-induced asthma, inform the teacher that symptoms will begin about five minutes after the exertion has finished and last for about half an hour.

Prevention

At home

Upon waking each morning, spend a moment or two before rising from bed gently stretching each leg and then each arm, imagining that you are making them at least twelve inches longer. Then stand by the bed and take a slow deep yoga breath, expanding the chest and forcing your shoulders back as you breathe. Mentally tell yourself that for the rest of the day you are going to walk tall, with chest out, and take slow deep breaths.

From time to time throughout the day, stop what you are doing and take a deliberate slow deep breath. This reminds the body that you are in charge, and prevents it from slipping back into old breathing habits.

Children at home

For young children who cannot master breathing techniques, a simple but effective method of improving breathing capacity, at the same time helping to clear the lungs of mucus, is bubble blowing. The old-fashioned bowl of thick soap and a clay pipe are all that is needed. A regular session during the tight chest period will help, whilst at the same time the child's subconscious will associate floating bubbles with chest relief. This can be used to good effect if, for instance, the child is having a difficult night. With his or her eyes closed, you encourage the child to visualize a mental picture of bubbles floating gently up. You will often encourage a relaxed chest and a relaxed sleep.

In the car

Driving to work is a good time to practise deep breathing and relaxation. Make sure that you have a fresh air vent open and not too much heating on, that your seat is properly adjusted so you sit reasonably erect, and not slumped with the chest pressing on the stomach. The hands should grip the steering wheel at the 'quarter to three' position: this means that your arms are comfortably extended, allowing your chest to expand more freely. Every four or five minutes you should take three or four 'yoga breaths' as you drive, and push your shoulders down as you breathe out each time. Mentally settle back and relax your mind, and do not allow other drivers to upset you. If somebody makes a silly mistake, pull back and let them 'get on with it'. In this way you should arrive at work in a calm and relaxed state which will set the pattern of the day.

At work

No matter what your work is, from office to factory floor, you can still follow a simple routine and repeat it frequently throughout the day. First you must try and arrive early each day, as a late start causes tension and stress. Preferably find a few minutes before you start, and at lunchtime, to attempt a short walk while using the breathing techniques. Mentally this is good for you as it reminds you how important you are, and it also disciplines the physical body. If your work is of a nature that requires absolute concentration, then you must not take the odd minute or two to relax, but you can switch on yoga breathing every few minutes and make sure your chest is expanding well and the shoulders are pushed back.

In the office it is usually much simpler to sit back in your chair from time to time and take one or two yoga breaths, close your eyes to visualize a picture of yourself striding healthily along a path. With regular application you will find to your surprise that you have attained a new image and you are striding through the office with shoulders back and chest out.

During pregnancy

Throughout the pregnancy it is important to retain a calm and tranquil state of mind; this will also help the baby who is sensitive to your moods. At least three or four times a day you should take time to lie on your back using a folded blanket on the floor and follow the relaxation and breathing routines. If you practise regularly throughout the pregnancy, you will find during the birth that your relaxation and breathing techniques become second nature, allowing easy breathing and a pain-free birth. This can be used to advantage even if you have a hospital birth.

Later the techniques will help you whilst feeding your baby, and also help to release the tensions of the day.

5
The world of herbs

Among the many alternative therapies used for the treatment of asthma, herbal medicine is perhaps the oldest. It has been discovered that early man had knowledge of the healing power of plants, and many animals and birds appear to have inherited a genetic knowledge of particular herbs and their healing properties.

Man has discovered over 750,000 different species of flowering plant on this planet, and history shows that many have been, and still are, employed as medicines throughout the civilized world as well as by the remotest 'primitive' tribes. These employ tribal witch doctors who continue to use the knowledge passed down over centuries of plant medicines to treat their people and animals. Despite the vast changes which have taken place to produce this modern scientific world, and the comparatively recent swing to chemical drugs, many people continue to use herbs as medicines, either preparing them in the home, or by consulting a medical herbalist. Many of the drugs that were formally used by doctors contained plant-based medicines, and even today many leading drugs are derived from plants. Did you know for instance that the heart drug *digoxin* is from digitalis, more commonly known as foxglove, that aspirin is derived from a species of willow, and that belladonna is still used in modern drugs?

And yet, despite the thousands of years of acquired knowledge, and although we know that a particular herb works for a certain condition, we do not always know why; on the other hand, orthodox medicine works on the principle of examining each drug and understanding the way in which it works. This does not necessarily make drugs safer to use; indeed, their side-effects have to a certain extent increased the popularity of herbal medicine.

Herbs have always been considered safe and gentle in their action and history proves this. However, it must be remembered that a plant may contain substances which, if taken in too strong a dose, may cause distressing effects. A plant is a living organism with a complex make-up: it may contain acids, sugars, alkaloids, starch, resins, vitamins, minerals and traces of metals. It is the presence of these ingredients which make a plant medicine active, and provides its healing action, but like many other 'safe' things on this earth, plants, if taken to excess, can be detrimental rather than beneficial.

In preparing a medicine to be used in the home, always follow the recommended method, as well as the suggested quantities of herb and fluid.

Also bear in mind that the medicinal value of a plant can be influenced by certain factors, such as the season in which it is picked, as well as the way in which it is prepared as a medicine. Do not attempt to make a 'stronger brew' in the belief that it will work better; remember it has taken thousands of years to acquire the knowledge of the safe and effective dose.

How to prepare herbs

There are numerous ways to make herbs into medicines, and they are all intended to achieve the same end, that of extracting the juice from the plant.

Some methods are reserved for the laboratory because some plants require special methods to extract from them their active principles, or because a more concentrated extraction is required. However for home use there are two rather simpler methods which have been used for many years called *infusion* and *decoction*: these need only the equipment that can be found in the average kitchen and are suitabe both for dried and fresh herbs.

Infusions

These preparations can be made from ground or bruised roots, bark, leaves or seeds, and flower heads. The method is very similar to making ordinary tea, and like tea it is best to use a glass or earthenware container. Simply pour boiling water over a measured amount of the herb, let it stand for half an hour, stirring occasionally. When cooled, the infusion is strained through a cloth and carefully stored in a cool place. It is always best to use a fresh infusion (not more than 24 hours old). Ideally, of course, each dose should be freshly made; however, this is not always practical, and it could prove rather wasteful if the herb was expensive.

An infusion will usually keep for 24 hours and can be bottled, or put into a jug and stored in the warmest part of the refrigerator, or in a dark, cool cupboard.

The usual quantity of herb used in an infusion is 1 oz (30g) to 1 pint (½ litre) of water. The dose varies from a tablespoonful to a wineglassful or a teacup.

Decoctions

These are made by pouring cold water upon the cut, bruised, or ground herb, the mixture being boiled for twenty minutes to half an hour, cooled, and strained. Roots and barks are best treated in this way as they need a longer period subjected to heat in order to release the active principles. It is also a way of making a stronger medicine from the herb, as decoctions are generally made from 1 oz (30g) of the herb to one and a half pints (¾ litre) of water, and the mixture gently boiled until a pint (½ litre) of the fluid remains.

The dose varies from two teaspoonfuls to one or two wineglasses.

Fresh herbs

Choose only vigorous, healthy-looking plants, and if you are picking the leaf remember the quality is better before the plant goes to seed. When gathering herbs observe the plant habit: for instance if a particular plant prefers the sun, then choose a plant which is growing in a sunny aspect. Likewise, if your herbal supplies are from a shade-loving plant, pick them from one that is actually growing in a shady place. This ensures that you have a better quality herb, which means that your medicine will also be of good quality.

Bruising and cutting

These are methods of preparing fresh picked herbs before using them for infusion or decoction.

Bruising is a method of breaking the surface of the herb, usually the root or bark, although the leaves can also be treated this way. The herb is placed in a mortar and pounded gently with a pestle, or the herb can be placed on a hard surface and gently pounded with the edge of a wooden rolling pin.

Cutting is usually applied to leaves, and it is simply done by cutting the leaves into smaller parts using a sharp knife or scissors. Both these methods are to help the extraction of the active principle within the plant during infusion or decoction.

Dried herbs

Sometimes the fresh herb is not available: either the season is wrong for picking, or the herb you require does not grow in your area, or your country. It is perfectly acceptable to use dried herbs in exactly the same way as you would fresh.

Supplies of these can be obtained from some health food shops, or sometimes a medical herbalist will be prepared to supply you with dried herbs or fluid extracts. In some towns can be found a shop that specializes in selling dried herbs, such as 'Culpepers'. Look in your local business directory or yellow pages for medical herbalists or herbal shops.

Drying your own herbs

Dried herbs are the most convenient way of keeping a supply of the herbs that you will need through the months when the fresh plant is not available. The fresh herb needs to be gathered as dry as possible, that is after the morning dew on them has been dried by the sun. The cut herbs should be hung in bunches upside down to dry, in the sun if possible. If not, hang them in a warm room in an area that has flowing air. When dry they should be hung in paper bags in a warm dry atmosphere.

Seed heads do not need a lot of drying, as nature has already commenced the process.

Before drying roots they should be examined for blemishes, and any with blemishes or parts that appear rotten should be rejected. Remember to choose your herbs just as if you were choosing vegetables from a supermarket shelf: choose only the best.

Preparation of roots

Roots should be washed, dried, and then roasted in an oven. When roasting is complete they should then be ground as you would coffee, and the ground root should then be kept in a well-sealed container, preferably in the dark.

Seed heads and leaves

Dried seed heads and dried leaves can be kept in well-sealed containers, or hung in paper bags. Both can be left attached to their stalks and used directly from the stalk.

Herbs and asthma

Over the centuries many herbs have been discovered that help the symptoms of asthma, but just as those symptoms can vary from person to person, so must the herb or herbs be chosen according to the symptoms.

Each herb has its own healing property. Some are soothing to the irritated air passages which cause a dry cough. Some have the ability to promote the breaking of tight mucus, whilst others have the ability to lift the mucus from the chest. One of the advantages of herbs is their ability to be mixed together, thereby making a medicine capable of treating a number of different symptoms.

The following list contains herbs that can be used for asthma in its different stages as well as some of the symptoms which precede or follow it. The list also contains some of the most used and valuable herbs employed today by the modern medical herbalist in treating the different types of asthma.

Some of the medical terms used to describe their individual actions on the human body are listed at the end of this chapter.

Herbal pharmacopoeia for asthma

Coltsfoot (*Tussilago farfara*) otherwise known as
Coughwort, Horsefoot or Foal's foot

A very common wild plant found in the British Isles. It has powerful expectorant as well as strong soothing qualities to the chest and lungs. The leaves or the flowers can be used to make a decoction, which is then sweetened with honey and taken in teacupful doses.

It is especially useful for elderly people who suffer intrinsic asthma as it aids in bringing up mucus which is often present in the lungs. It will also help relieve a tight chest and, if taken as a daily medicine, may prevent the next attack of bronchitis before it turns to asthma.

The dried leaves of this plant are used as a herbal tobacco and, when smoked, this appears to bring some relief to coughs and tight chests.

It can be bought in tablet form under the name 'Potter's Antibron tablets' which also contain euphorbia, pleurisy root and senega in their formula.

Chamomile (*Anthernis nobilis*) antispasmodic, sedative
and tonic

A much-used herb for many complaints, but for asthma in particular it works in several ways: its antispasmodic properties make it a useful remedy to be given during an asthma attack; its sedative properties act by calming the nerves; and its tonic properties promote a sense of well-being.

In all, it is a very useful herb for the asthmatic, but its main attraction lies in its healing record for children and babies. It can be given safely and frequently to ease difficult breathing, to calm anxiety and promote sleep. It is an excellent remedy also for toothache.

The flower is used to make an infusion which can be taken frequently in teacupful doses. The taste is pleasant, and it can be taken in place of tea or coffee as a relaxant.

For young children and babies a half ounce (15g) of the herb to 1 pint (½ litre) of water is recommended to make the infusion. This can then be sweetened and given frequently in teaspoonful doses.

Chamomile teabags are also available from health shops.

Euphorbia (*Euphorbia hirta*, or *Euphorbia pilulifere*)
otherwise known as Asthma-weed or Catshair
A very definite 'anti-asthmatic herb', able to bring prompt relief to paroxysmal asthma, by relieving spasm. For the chronic asthmatic, a regular dose before meals may help to prevent the asthma spasm occurring.

The infusion of a half ounce (15g) of herb in 1 pint (½ litre) of water is taken in tablespoon doses.

Golden Seal (*Hydrastis canadensis*) otherwise known as Orange or Yellow root
This is a most expensive but valuable herb, being employed for any condition that affects mucous membranes in the body. It is of particular value in both extrinsic and intrinsic asthma, having a cleansing and restorative effect on inflamed membrane, whilst its definite tonic properties help restore vitality and health.

The part used is the root and it is prepared as a decoction; the dose is one wineglassful before food.

Horehound (*Marrubium vulgare*)
This is a popular herb used for asthma, bronchitis, colds and catarrh. Unlike most herbs, it has a pleasant taste and is used frequently with hyssop to make a very soothing and powerful cough and catarrh treatment. Horehound is used widely in patent herbal cough medicines, often combined with aniseed.

An infusion can be made from 1 oz (30g) of each to 1 pint (½ litre) of water and taken in wineglassful doses frequently.

Liquorice (*Glycyrrhiza glabra*)
The root of the liquorice plant is a powerful medicine for the chest and lungs and is used frequently as a base when mixing herbs together as it forms an agreeable taste as well as being itself a chest medicine.

It can be prepared as an infusion to be used by itself as a medicine, or a decoction to make a more powerful medicine as a base for a mixture.

The dose of infusion is a wineglassful for adults, and a dessertspoonful for children.

Lobelia (*Lobelia inflata*) otherwise known as Indian
Tobacco or Pukeweed
This is one of nature's most valuable herbs for the asthmatic and it is used widely for its amazing antispasmodic
action. It is to be found in most formulae for asthma and
chest mixtures and is both expectorant, and antispasmodic, as well as stimulant, in large doses it acts as an
emetic, hence its name 'pukeweed'.

It has both expectorant and antispasmodic properties
which work very quickly. Mucus is lifted from the chest
after just one dose of the infusion, and a single dose has
been known to bring instant relief from asthma spasm.

It should be taken regularly while there is cough,
catarrh, or wheezing, and it can be sipped throughout an
asthma attack.

The infusion, of 1 oz (30g) of powdered herb, to 1 pint
(½ litre) water, is taken in half to one wineglassful doses.

It can also be purchased in tablet form from health
shops under the brand name 'Gerard House Lobelia
Compound Tablets'.

Mullein (*Verbascum thapsus*) also known as Blanket Herb
or Lady's Foxglove
Grows in Britain, and flowers in late summer.

Both leaves and flowers have a beneficial effect on
asthma, and the infusion can be taken in wineglassful
doses three times daily as a regular treatment, or every
hour if the asthma is bad.

Nettle (*Urtica dioica*) Stinging nettle
This is considered a common weed, and a great deal of
effort and money is spent trying to rid the garden of it.
However, as always nature is wise and provides its most
useful herbs in great quantities and the nettle is no
exception.

The seeds of the nettle are the part of the herb used for
asthma, and are prepared as an infusion which is
extremely valuable for relieving wheezing and shortness
of breath. It is also a useful herb for a troublesome cough.
It provides a valuable source of iron, for which the young
tops are picked and cooked like spinach. The dose is a
wineglassful 3 times daily.

Red Clover (*Trefolium pratense*) otherwise known as
Trefoil or Purple Clover
This extremely common plant to Britain is an excellent
remedy for spasmodic and bronchial coughs as well as
whooping cough. The method of preparing is by infusion
which may safely be taken frequently; I would suggest a
wineglassful for adults every hour when the asthma or
bronchitis is bad, a tablespoonful every hour for children
between 7 and 14 years old, and a teaspoonful for babies
and up to 7 years old. Sweeten with honey if necessary to
make it more drinkable for the young.

Violet (*Viola odorata*) otherwise known as Blue Violet or
Sweet Violet
It possesses strong antiseptic and expectorant properties,
and both the leaves and the flowers can be used. The
flowers have the stronger expectorant properties, whilst
the leaves have been used successfully in the treatment of
cancer.
    The leaf or flower is prepared by infusion and the dose
is a wineglassful three times daily.

Aromatic herbs

The herbs that come under this category contain volatile
oils which give off strong vapours. It is these vapours
which are particularly beneficial to the asthmatic. When
breathed in they help to release tightness and wheezing
in the chest, and the essential oils can be stored for long
periods and retain their power to release vapours when
warmed. The oils can be used to massage into the chest
and back and the heat of the body will ensure a slow
continuous release of the vapours.
    The oils also have a secondary beneficial action which
is their ability to produce either a stimulating, relaxing, or
toning effect when massaged into the skin. A few drops
of some of these oils are sometimes added to a herbal
mixture, because when taken internally as a medicine,
they have a warming, relaxing, and disinfecting action on
the inflamed mucous membrane of the air passages.
    During the process of infusion most aromatic herbs
release a certain amount of their essential oil and this can
be smelled in the steam. This steam, because of the oil it

contains, also has a medicinal action. This means that an infusion can be used to good effect by putting dried or fresh aromatic herbs into a large basin of hot water and breathing in the fumes with a towel over the head and basin.

You can also use a few drops of the distilled essential oils in the same way. The oil is very much stronger than the infusion and should be used cautiously when adding to mixtures – a single drop is often quite sufficient in a half to a pint of fluid (¼–½ litre).

Eucalyptus (*Eucalyptus globas*)   The leaf of the eucalyptus tree produces an extremely warming and volatile oil which makes an excellent chest rub. This is a valuable herb, having antiseptic, antispasmodic and stimulant qualities. The dried or the fresh leaves can be used to prepare an infusion for inhaling, or a few drops of oil of eucalyptus can be used in the hot water in place of leaves. It is best known for its antiseptic properties which are very effective. A drop or two can be added to a warm infusion of any other herbs that are being taken, or a cup of hot water with a little sugar or honey and two drops of the oil can be sipped frequently during an asthma attack. It is equally useful as a rub or inhalation for bronchitis.

Thyme   A common culinary herb, which is valuable for most asthmatics, it is tonic, antispasmodic and antiseptic. Its antiseptic properties are particularly useful to intrinsic asthma sufferers and, if taken regularly through the winter, may help to prevent an infection. The dose is a wineglass of the infusion taken frequently, or one or two drops of the distilled oil in a cup of hot sweetened water taken two or three times daily.

Marjoram   There are two species of this plant: the variety which is most useful has the Latin name *Origanum vulgare*. It has soothing properties which will help during an attack when its properties can be enhanced by adding a little honey to the hot infusion and sipping frequently.

It is prepared as an infusion, and the dose is a wineglass two or three times daily.

Romany cough and asthma remedy

1 oz (30g) of Liquorice root
1 oz (30g) of Coltsfoot
1 fresh lemon
Honey
3 pints (1½ litres) of water

Preparation
Simmer the liquorice root in three pints of water until it is reduced to one pint (½ litre), add the Coltsfoot and the sliced lemon. Stir well, strain, add honey to taste and take a wineglassful frequently.

Preventative asthma mixture

Chamomile 1 oz (30g)
Euphorbia 1 oz (30g)
Horehound 1 oz (30g)
Lobelia 1 oz (30g)
Mullein 1 oz (30g)

Preparation
Infuse in 1 pint (½ litre) of boiling water. When cool, strain and bottle. Take 1 tablespoonful in a little hot water and honey daily before meals.

Bronchitis and asthma mixture

Coltsfoot 1 oz (30g)
Chamomile 1 oz (30g)
Golden Seal 1 oz (30g)
Mullein 1 oz (30g)
Red Clover 1 oz (30g)
Liquorice 1 oz (30g)

Preparation
Add the above ingredients to one and half pints of water (¾ litre) and make a decoction. Strain, and add two pounds (1 kg) of sugar, gently heat and stir without boiling until the sugar is completely dissolved. The syrup can then be taken as a tablespoonful dose 3 times daily.

Asthma chest rub

A very effective chest rub to relieve spasm and open the air passages during an asthma attack. Mix together a few drops each of the following oils:

Oil of Eucalyptus
Lavender oil
Linseed oil
Oil of Pine

After warming the oils, massage gently into the chest and throat, and repeat every 2 or 3 hours until relief is obtained.

Asthma vapour bath

Eucalyptus
Lavender
Rosemary
Thyme
Pine

Take three ounces (90g) of each of the above and infuse into one pint of boiling water. When cooled, the infusion can be added to a hot bath to be taken before bedtime.

A few drops of the essential oil from each of these plants can be used in the bath instead of the infusion.

Most of the essential oils mentioned can be obtained in small quantities from chemists or health shops.

Many of the valuable herbs which grow in Britain can be obtained in seed form which are available from most garden centres. Even the smallest garden can find room for growing herbs, and they even grow well in pots, or window boxes.

Some of the aromatic herbs grown in a window box or pot on the kitchen sill will provide some relief to an asthma sufferer simply from the gentle aroma they give off.

Glossary of medical terms

Antispasmodic. Preventing or curing spasm.
Antiseptic. Counteracts sepsis by destroying bacteria.

Detergent. Cleansing.

Deobstruent. Clearing away obstructions by opening the natural passages of the body.

Emetic. Herbs which cause vomiting.

Expectorant. Promoting expectoration and removing secretions from the bronchial tubes.

Pectoral. Used in connection with drugs used internally for affections of the chest and lungs.

Sedative. Drugs which calm nervous excitement or tension.

Tonic. Substances which give tone to the body producing a feeling of well-being.

Case history of Mr A

Many years ago I met in the course of my clinical practice an old man who used to smoke the most foul-smelling home-made cigarettes. He was a sprightly soul always full of good humour and tall stories. He confided to me that as a child he had been a chronic asthmatic, and that on several occasions his parents had despaired of his survival. He was born in 1895 when inhalers were unknown and emergency treatment consisted of inhaling the steam from Friar's Balsam.

I pointed out to him that with his history of asthma the last thing he should be doing was smoking. With a twinkle in his eye he told me that he was smoking the very thing that had cured his asthma! It was the herb coltsfoot. He told me that when he was five years old his mother had met an old lady in the park who had noticed how badly the boy was breathing. The old lady had then taken her to a small meadow nearby, and by a stream had pointed out a small shrub covered in yellow flowers; this was coltsfoot. She had picked the flower heads and told the mother to put one ounce in a saucepan with two pints of water, to be boiled gently until reduced to one pint. She was instructed to strain the liquid and add to it one tablespoonful of honey. This was to be given to the child frequently a teacupful at a time. The old lady also told her that when the flowers of the coltsfoot faded that they would be followed by the leaves which would be equally effective, and that in the winter when the leaves disappeared the root could be used.

So successful did the treatment prove that within a year the boy was almost without asthma, although each winter his mother continued with the treatment. His health continued to improve, and when he reached his teens he was well enough to be accepted into the navy. It was during his naval service that he learnt of a cheap tobacco that was made from a shredded herb. When he discovered it was coltsfoot it had seemed to complete a cycle and he had smoked it ever since; he boasted that he had never had an asthma attack in 70 years.

Case history of Miss Jennifer C

Jennifer C was seven years old, and she had suffered asthma and eczema since she was a baby. When I first examined her it was because the eczema was causing a lot of discomfort and her skin was raw and bleeding in places where she had scratched for relief. Her mother was worried because her general health was suffering from lack of sleep, her appetite was poor, and she had become very low in herself. She was tearful and had bouts of irritability. She was prescribed red clover and chamomile, an infusion to be given every two hours with honey. An ointment made from marigolds called *calendula* was prescribed to soothe the skin. Within a week Jennifer's mother reported a definite improvement in her skin and she appeared to be far happier in herself. At this stage medication would normally have been drastically reduced, but because of her history of asthma and eczema it was decided to continue the infusion for several more weeks. The decision proved correct and she continued to improve both in skin and lungs. Eventually she was taking only a dose of the infusion at night and no longer needed her calendula ointment. I saw Jennifer a year later and she was growing into a lovely girl; she had no eczema or asthma and was showing much promise at school.

- Red clover had been chosen for its blood cleansing properties as well as its beneficial action on the lungs; this with chamomile for its nerve-soothing properties proved to be a constitutional treatment for Jennifer.

Case history of Mr D

When Mr D first consulted me he was 55 years old, and had been forced into early retirement from a job in the City due to chronic bronchitic asthma. It was a great effort for him to walk the few steps from my waiting room to the consulting room, where he eventually sat gasping for breath. He was not overweight; indeed he was of quite a slim build and there was no history of asthma in his family. He did however have a history as a child of recurring chest infections, which through his teens had seemed to improve. It was when he went to work in the City that his chest began to worsen. When questioned, he admitted that the traffic fumes caused him much aggravation. On further questioning it was found that he followed a bad diet, and frequently had quick business lunches eaten standing in a smoke-filled bar.

His asthma was diagnosed as intrinsic, and he was given dietary advice and prescribed golden seal, euphorbia, and lobelia, in a syrup with root ginger. He was advised to follow some breathing exercises and to attempt a little daily exercise which would help clear the loosened mucus from the chest. Within three months he was showing distinct signs of improvement, and was then prescribed red clover, mullein, euphorbia and coltsfoot to be taken three times daily as an infusion. This helped to prevent the recurring chest infections through the winter months and to the best of my knowledge he has continued to enjoy relatively good health for the past five years.

6
Homoeopathy

Understanding and using the tiny dose

The secret of the 'tiny dose' has been known and used for centuries, it is believed that the great Paracelsus and Hippocrates, 'the father of medicine' had knowledge of the dilution. The name homoeopathy is coined from the Greek, and means *like – disease*; in fact, the basic philosophy underlying the treatment by homoeopathic medicine is 'like cures like'. This is based upon the theory that diseases are curable by those drugs which produce effects on the body similar to the symptoms caused by the disease. In administering the drugs, the theory is also held that their effect is increased by giving them in minute doses obtained by diluting them to an extreme degree.

The term 'drug' is not often used in homoeopathy: we prefer to call our medicines 'remedies', this is simply to separate them from the drugs employed by orthodox medicine which are derived mostly from chemical origins. Homoeopathic remedies are derived from a range of substances, which may vary from plants to minerals, and from animal substances to deadly poisons. All are rendered harmless by the process of dilution.

The homoeopathic dilution

Samuel Hahnemann, a German doctor, re-discovered the use of the 'tiny dose' and introduced its concepts in 1810. He also compiled a *materia medica* (a dictionary of symptoms).

Hahnemann evolved a method of mixing, diluting and shaking which he called succussion. The result of this was a powerful preparation which he called a potency. The means of producing the base for the medicine if it was of plant or mineral extraction was to grind the chosen substance with a pestle and mortar. It was then rendered into liquid form by dissolving in a mixture of alcohol and water, producing what was called the *mother tincture*. Some substances already liquid by nature can be directly dissolved with alcohol and water to form the mother tincture.

The mother tincture was then diluted methodically, the diluent often being a similar mixture of alcohol and water. One drop of mother tincture in 10 drops of diluent is called 1x dilution (from x = 10). One drop of mother tincture in 99 drops of diluent is called a 1c (from c = 100). By a further series of dilution and succussion, higher potencies are produced which go up to any level required. The principal is, the greater the degree of dilution, the more powerful the medicine becomes.

It is this apparent paradox which confuses many people and causes the most criticism from orthodox sources. None the less, Hahnemann proved his theories of the tiny dose by producing the cures, and today there are thousands of people who will bear testimony to the continuing effectiveness of the homoeopathic dilution, often when all other forms of treatment have failed.

Choosing a remedy

For the asthmatic homoeopathy offers a safe and gentle method of treatment which seeks not only to help the immediate symptoms, but also to encourage the body to produce a cure. There is a saying in homoeopathy: 'Every disease is curable, but not every patient is.' This implies a cause of the illness in some patients which is beyond the knowledge of medical science. The principle of stimulating the body to heal itself has sometimes produced a cure in so-called 'incurable' cases; this is because the power of nature holds many secrets which have yet to be discovered. Homoeopathy seeks to unleash that power and encourage a return to harmony thereby overcoming the 'disease' condition. Until the causes are discovered the human race will have to continue acknowledging the existence of some diseases which to it are 'incurable' because this is as far as our knowledge extends. Homoeopathy, looking beyond the disease, tries to stimulate the 'vital force' or 'healing power' of the body by the administration of extremely tiny doses of varying substances.

The remedy is selected after studying the symptoms which the disease is producing, and then seeking the remedy which in its crude state would have produced 'similar' symptoms in a healthy person. Many people mistakenly believe that homoeopathy works on the same principle as inoculation. This is not true. Inoculation works on the principle of 'identicals' – that is, the vaccine administered is of the disease that you are trying to gain protection from. Homoeopathy, on the other hand, works on the principle of 'similars' in which the symptoms of the disease need to be similar or match closely the symptoms of the remedy. It is important to understand that, when considering the choice of remedy, other factors than the disease are taken into account.

The qualified homoeopathic practitioner chooses a remedy after an extensive questionnaire has been answered which covers every aspect of the patient. The symptoms, no matter how trivial they may appear are recorded, the patient's build and colouring are noted, as well as habits and the mental and emotional category they come under. This information is then applied to a *materia medica*, which is a book or series of books in which are recorded hundreds of symptoms together with the remedies which the symptoms indicate.

For each symptom the materia medica will often list dozens of remedies. *It is the remedy which appears most often and fits the symptom pattern most closely which is ultimately chosen.*

This method of selecting the remedy confuses many people when trying to use homoeopathy in the home. The most common complaint is that every remedy seems to contain some of the symptoms. This of course is true, but the factor which simplifies the selection of the remedy is the colouring and build of the patient.

This narrows the field of selection considerably be-cause homoeopathy has remedies for fat people, thin people, fair and blue eyed, or dark hair and brown eyed people.

Pulsatilla is a remedy which suits 'fair haired, blue eyed' people, Sepia is for 'dark haired, slim females', whilst Calc. Carb. suits chubby children with sleep problems, and Sulphur is indicated for 'untidy people with skin or chest troubles'.

For home use you can obtain a much reduced materia medica. This will list only one or two important symptoms, together with build or colouring which will enable the home user to find the remedy quickly and safely.

Such a materia medica is published by Nelsons and can be obtained from homoeopathic dispensaries, chemists and health stores.

Asthma prevention

The general text of this book is how to treat your asthma, but the underlying philosophy of all medicine should be in **prevention**.

Preventing intrinsic asthma

To the intrinsic asthma sufferer autumn and winter are the times of the year to be feared, due to a tendency in the intrinsic asthmatic toward chest infections, as well as colds and flu. Often these infections can lead to asthma and so should be avoided at all costs. By seeking to prevent infection the asthma sufferer increases the chances of avoiding the recurring aggravations of the condition.

Precautions in the winter

Orthodox medicine as yet has no answer to the common cold, or to influenza, and admits that each year by the time it has developed a vaccine for the previous strain of influenza, a new one has developed.

Homoeopathy, on the other hand, offers specific remedies for the prevention and treatment of the common cold and influenza, and the remedies are perfectly safe to use for babies and the elderly.

The common cold

Homoeopathic remedy: Nat Mur 30c. (*Natrum Muriaticum*)

Symptoms The common cold usually begins with a sore throat, or runny eyes and nose, or tickling in the nose with sneezing. These symptoms usually commence in the first 12 hours of the infection, and successful treatment means treating the very first tickle or sneeze. At the first indication of the symptoms the remedy should be taken and continued until all symptoms have cleared.

Prevention Always remember that prevention is better than cure. This is particularly true of the common cold which brings misery and discomfort to hundreds of thousands each year. If you have had contact with anyone showing symptoms of the common cold, you should take one dose of Nat Mur 30c immediately followed by two further doses at four to six hourly intervals. If you work in an environment among a large number of people it may be useful to take a preventative treatment as an insurance against infection. This is effected by taking three doses of Nat Mur 30c at 12 hourly intervals, and repeating the three doses every seven days throughout the winter months.

Treatment This should begin as soon as possible after the first symptom is experienced. Nat Mur should be taken in the first 12 hours at two hourly intervals, reducing to every four hours as the symptoms subside, but if the cold has developed past the 12 hour stage, I would suggest taking Gelsemium as well as Nat Mur, the remedies to be taken at the same frequency but half an hour apart.

Influenza

Homoeopathic remedy: Gelsemium 200c.
The influenza virus has shown remarkable agility over the past decade by changing its symptom pattern frequently. One year it manifests in joint pains and headaches, the next year it may produce a terrible cough followed by a chronic mucus buildup in the upper respiratory tract. Always it is accompanied by debility.

During the past 20 years of clinical practice I have noticed a tendency for the symptoms of influenza to linger for longer periods. This may indicate that the strains are becoming stronger, or our resistance weaker. Each strain has been given its own name, and they are capable of producing epidemics which in the past have killed thousands of people. Elderly people are particularly vulnerable.

Medical science can often predict where the next epidemic is going to attack and orthodox as well as homoeopathic medicine has produced vaccines which contain the strains of the previous flu viruses.

In many cases these are effective, but despite the surface symptoms changing, my clinical observation suggests that the essential influenza virus remains the same, and I believe the traditional treatment which has always used Gelsemium is still the best and most effective remedy.

Treatment   One dose should be taken every two hours during the first symptoms, and reduced to every four hours when the symptoms begin to subside.

Prevention   Take one dose every 12 hours for three doses. This should be repeated every seven days during the period you are at risk. The remedy may be taken together with the common cold treatment.

Preventative treatment should be taken if you have been in contact with somebody infected with the virus but are not experiencing symptoms, or if you simply want to insure against flu throughout the winter months.

Not long ago a flu epidemic was raging and my dispensary was approached by the headmaster of a large private boarding school for preventative treatment for his pupils and staff. Gelsemium 200c was prescribed and five thousand tablets were prepared to be given one dose every 24 hours. He reported three months later that not one of his staff or pupils had contracted symptoms of flu.

Bronchitis

Homoeopathic remedy: Aconite. (*Aconitum Napellus*)
This is one of the inherent diseases of Great Britain,

brought on mainly by the damp, misty weather which we as an island experience during the winter months. To the asthmatic, bronchitis is to be avoided at all costs, as it can often lead to weeks of tight chest and wheezing symptoms, sometimes developing into full-blown bronchitic asthma. Recurring bouts of this produce a gradual and progressive weakening of the 'vital force' which in turn produces an increasing susceptability.

Prevention   There is no specific homoeopathic remedy for the prevention of bronchitis, but a general recommendation is to take the cold and flu prevention treatments throughout the winter months plus a supplement such as cod liver oil. Also ensure regular hot meals, and a warm, dry atmosphere to try and avoid chest infections.

Treatment   Aconite; Carbo Veg.; Drosera; Ipecac.; Kali Bich.; Phosphorus.

In severe cases of bronchitic asthma when breathing is particularly bad, a dose of Aconite 200c given every 4 hours can prove beneficial.

Preventing extrinsic asthma

The prevention of extrinsic asthma presents a more difficult task than that of intrinsic asthma because the causes are so variable. A large number of causes have been isolated to certain foods which contain gluten, white sugar, moulds or additives which are identified by E numbers. Industrial emissions, as well as smog from car exhausts, pollens and dust can cause asthma. The logical approach to prevention would appear to lie in the avoidance of known allergens, but as most of these are airborne this would be virtually impossible. Therefore the basis of treatment must lie in two areas. One is to identify the allergens and the other is to attempt to provoke an immunity in the body which will prevent the allergic reaction.

There are a number of ways to identify the allergen, and these are explained in Chapter 10. Once identified, the patient can then undergo desensitization treatment.

This is achieved homoeopathically by giving doses of the allergen in high dilutions.

Many of these can be purchased ready prepared. Ainsworth's Homoeopathic Pharmacy in London produce an impressive range of 300 different allergen remedies, from aftershave to wheat gluten. The range also includes 23 individual E numbers from food additives, as well as house dust mite, mixed grass pollens, grass mowings, mixed moulds, and a range of individual pollens including rose, orange blossom, and rape seed.*

Asthma in the spring and summer

For many extrinsic asthma sufferers the spring and summer months are the worst, because this is when the pollens from grasses, trees and flowers are airborne. I have selected a few of the most used homoeopathic remedies for the symptoms of summer allergies, which can give considerable relief to many of the distressing symptoms such as tight breathing, irritating coughs, and chronic mucus production.

- Mixed Pollen
- Arsenicum Alb.
- Mixed Grasses
- Carbo Veg.
- Drosera

- Kali Bich.
- Phosphorus
- Ipecac.
- Pulsatilla
- Sulphur

Asthma and pregnancy

Many women will say that they never felt better than when they were pregnant, and indeed some women will tell you that during pregnancy their asthma subsided. Unfortunately there is a small percentage of women, usually those who suffer severe asthma, for whom pregnancy is a nightmare. The reason is that a number of asthma 'drugs' are not recommended in the first few months of pregnancy and for some this can lead to weeks or months of hospitalization due to uncontrolled attacks. There is also a risk that blood oxygen levels may fall dangerously low if severe asthma attacks are allowed to

* A recent report linked a marked increase in the number of farms now growing rape seed with an increase in the number of asthma sufferers.

recur, and this is not only dangerous to the pregnant woman, but could also be potentially harmful to the unborn baby.

If you are suffering severe recurring asthma attacks during your pregnancy, contact your doctor – do not allow them to steadily worsen.

However, because homoeopathic remedies are safe to use during pregnancy, the asthmatic who suffers mild to medium asthma may well consider using some of the remedies outlined. But if you suffer severe asthma it would be advisable to consider consulting a homoeopathic practitioner who would be able to monitor your treatment throughout the pregnancy.

In planning the management of your asthma during pregnancy, it is wise to prepare a programme that will take into account your needs at the different stages of the pregnancy.

It should contain natural supplements, a good diet, and exercise as well as breathing and relaxation techniques.

You should also have a 'pregnancy first aid kit' of homoeopathic remedies which should contain:

- Aconite for tight breathing.
- Bryonia for asthma on exertion.
- Chamomile for restful sleep.
- Caulophyllum for easy birth.
- Nat. Mur. for rhinitus and colds.
- Sepia for postnatal depression.
- Symphoricarpus Racemosa for morning sickness.

Hyperventilation of pregnancy

Some women can experience a type of 'false asthma' during pregnancy, caused by increased levels of the hormone progesterone. This has the effect of stimulating the breathing pattern which may give rise to a feeling of shortness of breath. This is not a worsening of the asthma condition, but a form of 'hyperventilation' which would usually be treated with sedatives by the doctor. However as these are not recommended to be prescribed during pregnancy I would suggest taking homoeopathic aconite to relieve the symptoms.

Vasomotor rhinitis of pregnancy

Another aggravation that may arise as a result of pregnancy is rhinitis or severe nasal congestion. This is known as 'vasomotor rhinitis of pregnancy'. The congestion often starts around the first three months of pregnancy. Again the usual drugs for rhinitis cannot be given but homoeopathic Nat. Mur., the 'common cold remedy', will control the rhinitis safely and effectively.

Homoeopathic treatment for babies and children

Of all the therapies outlined in this book, homoeopathy offers the safest treatment for babies and young children. It should of course form a part of an all-embracing care programme in which diet and environmental care also play a role, but the homoeopathic remedy will give the worried parents a safe and speedy method of relieving many of the distressing symptoms of childhood asthma.

There are also stages of growth through which a child goes that produce periods of increased susceptibility to asthma.

I have chosen the two periods to treat that appear to cause concern to most mothers: they are teething, and starting school.

Teething problems

Most babies experience a certain amount of difficulty during the teething period, some more than others. Apart from the usual discomfort experienced from the teeth coming through, many babies can run high temperatures and suffer from runny noses, as well as picking up coughs and chest infections, and some may experience convulsions or fits during this stage of their growth.

It is worth noting that if a baby is going to have a tendency to asthma, it is during the teething period that it is most likely to show. The two main remedies which are excellent for both asthma and teething are belladonna and chamomile.

Starting school

For both mothers and children, starting school is a very difficult time. The child can be anxious and tearful as he or she has to learn to deal with situations unaided for the first time, as well as learning to get along with a classful of others. Children also have a tendency to worry inwardly if they have problems; for instance a common problem is not understanding the instructions of the teacher, or the class may have a bully and the child is 'picked on'.

The asthmatic child can get very 'uptight' in these situations as for the first time in their life he/she has to stand up for him- or herself.

Exam nerves are another area of concern for most parents, not least the parent of an asthmatic, for often the nerves will manifest in an asthma attack.

Homoeopathy offers the following remedies for the asthmatic in all these situations:

Aconite; argent nit.; bryonia; gelsemium; silica.

Whooping cough

Whooping cough is a disease which most parents dread, not least the parents of an asthmatic baby. Whooping cough can lead to serious after-effects and in rare cases has proved fatal. On the other hand, the orthodox vaccine is also known to have possible serious side-effects in rare cases. Most parents with asthmatic babies do wisely agree to the inoculation offered by their general practitioner. However, in some cases, particularly if there is a history in the family of epilepsy or fits, or if the child has suffered convulsions, it is deemed unwise to give this injection due to the risk of brain damage.

If your child has been refused the injection, or if you are among those parents caught between the dreadful horns of a dilemma, unsure on the one hand whether to take the risk of possible side-effects, and on the other worried that if you do not agree you may be responsible for your child contracting the disease, homoeopathy offers a vaccine.

Homoeopathy has used its own whooping cough vaccine for a number of years and it has proved very successful. Obviously there cannot be a guarantee with any vaccine, orthodox or alternative, but from my experience of the hundreds I have prescribed for, to my knowledge only one child contracted whooping cough, and that was a very mild dose.

The remedy used is Pertussin 30c.* This is a nosode, which means it is a remedy prepared from the virus. Three doses are given at 12 hourly intervals, and this is repeated every four weeks for a period of three months. Immunity must not be presumed until the course is completed.

The vaccine is not recommended for babies under 12 weeks old, but do remember that during the breast feeding period the baby derives a natural immunity from its mother.

To ensure protection for the baby during the 12-week treatment period, it is suggested that any member of the family who has been in contact with whooping cough should take a dose of Drosera 12c night and morning for three days following the contact.

Treating whooping cough in the asthmatic child
Homoeopathic remedies:
Aconite; bryonia; carbo veg.; drosera; ipecac.

The following *materia medica* outlines some of the popular remedies for the relief of many of the symptoms of asthma as well as related symptoms such as anxiety, sleeplessness, debility, and catarrh. It is representative of only a fraction of the vast number of remedies available, but it will enable the reader to choose quickly and efficiently from the selected remedies mentioned in this chapter.

Homoeopathic types

As a brief guide to the use of the *materia medica* the following homoeopathic pictures may be useful:

* Pertussin can only be obtained on prescription from a homoeopathic practitioner.

Executive asthma

For the busy executive who starts his day with a hurried breakfast before catching the train to the office, who cannot find a seat on the train or a taxi at the other end; who deals with a thousand and one items during the morning and then entertains his clients to a pub lunch, who works on the train home; who needs a few stiff drinks to unwind, and then suffers indigestion or asthma through the night:

● **Nux Vomica** is the remedy.

Asthma at the kitchen sink

For the tired-out housewife with a demanding family, whose day starts by preparing breakfast and at the same time getting husband off to work, packing sandwiches for school, and feeding the ever-crying baby; who has not looked seriously at herself in a mirror for months because she has lost interest, and who is worried at the way she has begun to shout at the children:

● **Sepia** is the remedy.

Asthma and puberty

For the girl whose moods are as changeable as an April day, who dissolves into tears at the slightest criticism but can be happy and laughing a minute later; who worries because she hasn't begun her periods, or they have started and are extremely painful; who suffers much catarrh, but whose asthma is always better in the open air:

● Consider **Pulsatilla**.

The boy for whom puberty is a torture of spots, boils, and greasy hair; who perspires profusely on head, hands and feet; who is beset with inner anxieties, and constantly worries about not succeeding; who is the bullied and never the bully, whose moods drive everyone in the family frantic:

● The remedy is **Silica**.

Asthma and flying

For the asthmatic who gets 'uptight' at the very thought of air travel, who suffers claustrophobic asthma, and gets embarrassing 'nervous stomachs', who wheezes and chokes at the very thought of a stage appearance:

● **Argent Nit**. is the remedy.

Asthma and the elderly

For the elderly person whose asthma has caused a problem of overweight due to lack of exercise; whose every movement is slow and accompanied by wheezing and breathlessness; who punctuates each spoken word with a laboured breath; who is always pale and cold and yet needs to be fanned or sit near an open window:

● Consider **Carbo Veg**.

Materia medica for asthmatics

General instructions

Unless specifically stated the 6c or 12c potency is recommended. The dose is two tablets for adults and one tablet for babies or small children.

Frequency of dose should be:

Acute conditions, i.e. those that appear rapidly: one dose every hour for five or six doses, then reduce to one dose three times a day before or between meals.

Chronic conditions, i.e. those that are well established: one dose three times a day before or between meals until relief is obtained. Thereafter, one dose daily reducing to one dose weekly when all symptoms subside.

If any aggravation of symptoms is experienced while taking the medication, stop the medication. If the medication appeared to be helping before the aggravation, commence medication again only if original symptoms reappear.

Always store your homoeopathic remedies in a cool, dark place, away from strong smells.

Aconite (*aconitum napellus*)
● Symptoms appear suddenly, can be violent and brief.
● Exposure to cold wind and draughts.
● Very dry tight cough.
● Asthma spasm. Tight chest which worsens with anxiety.
● Anxiety, restlessness, fear, grief.
● Temperature with thirst.

- Aggravations: Around midnight. In a warm room or tobacco smoke. In cold winds.

Argent nit. (*argentum nitricum*)
- Chronic hoarseness. Suffocative cough as if a hair in the throat.
- Asthma brought on by fear or apprehension.
- Cannot breathe in a room full of people.
- Asthma with acidity. Dyspepsia with wind, which is worsened from nervousness.
- Nervous stomach, diarrhoea from nerves. Vomiting from nerves.
- Headaches. Fear of heights, claustrophobia, stage nerves.
- Nerves are the keynote to prescribing this remedy. Asthma accompanied with anxiety before a public appearance.
- Asthma before or during exams. Asthma from air travel.

Arsen. alb. (*arsenicum album*)
- Suits very tidy, fastidious, intelligent people.
- Asthma always better if patient kept warm. Symptoms worse between 2 and 3 a.m.
- Asthma with restlessness, fear and anxiety.
- Thirst, but will only sip fluids.
- Asthma at night; must have head raised to sleep. Cannot lie down for fear of suffocation.
- Asthma worse at midnight. Suffocative catarrh. Dry cough, worse after midnight and from lying on back.
- Dry skin, loss of weight. Chronic tiredness.

Belladonna (*atropa belladonna*)
- Asthma with bright, flushed face. High temperature.
- Throbbing headaches. Worse from the least jar or noise.
- Asthma with teething problems in babies. Grinding of teeth.
- Barking cough. Whooping cough. Moaning at every breath.
- Asthma with dry, hacking cough.
- Cannot bear to be touched. Cannot bear noise.

- Skin is dry and burning hot. Glands swollen and tender.

Bryonia (*bryonia alba*)
- Patient is intensely irritable and thirsty.
- Bursting, splitting headache.
- Chestiness, colds go down on to chest. Dry chest.
- Asthma with dry painful cough. Must sit up at night with asthma.
- Tough mucus deep in throat. Desire to take frequent deep breaths.
- Asthma symptoms worse from movement, and warmth. Better from rest.
- Asthma is better sitting with knees up.

Carbo veg. (*carbo vegetabilis*)
- Asthma in old people with lowered vitality. Breathing very shallow, must be fanned and have windows open.
- Asthma in persons who have never fully recovered from a previous illness.
- Chronic burping, and flatulence. Aversion to milk, meat and fatty food. Spasmodic asthma with gagging and vomiting of mucus.
- Wheezing and rattling in chest. First stages of whooping cough.

Caulophyllum (*caulophyllum thalictroides*)
One of the main functions of this remedy is to promote an easy birth, but it also relieves asthma during the final months of pregnancy.

Therefore if taken daily during the last four weeks of pregnancy it will perform the dual role of easy breathing and easy birth. Potency 30c. Dose 2 tablets daily.

Chamomile (*chamomilla*)
- Sensitive; irritable; thirsty.
- Asthma with whining restlessness. The child can't bear things, wants them, then throws them away. Wants to be picked up, then no sooner is this done, cries to be put down. Peevish disposition, nothing pleases.
- Toothache. Gums inflamed and red.

- Asthma with watery diarrhoea, can be greenish in teething babies.
- Colic. Thirst for cold water or acid drinks.
- Sleepless and restless at night with asthma.
- Asthma with catarrh, hoarseness, tenacious mucus in the throat.
- Asthma with dry cough, chiefly in the evening and at night in bed.
- Asthma with wheezing and rattling, made worse from anger.
- This remedy can be prescribed frequently, a dose every half hour if needed for acute cases of asthma or teething.

Drosera (sundew)
- Asthma with chronic dry coughs. The strain of coughing produces vomiting.
- Whooping cough. Annoying, tickling coughs in children only coming on in bed. Deep, hoarse voice.
- Asthma when speaking. Asthma that has not responded to other treatment.

Gelsemium (yellow jasmine)
- Influenza. Muscular weakness. Debility.
- Dull, heavy headaches. Vertigo.
- Sneezing with fullness at root of nose.
- Acute bronchitis. Feeling of weight on chest.
- Bronchial asthma. Asthma from fear/apprehension.
- Diarrhoea from emotional excitement, or fright or bad news.

Ipecacuana
- Persistent nausea and vomiting.
- Asthma with constant constriction in the chest.
- Yearly attacks of difficult breathing. Chronic bronchitis.
- Asthma with cough which is incessant and violent with every breath.
- Suffocative asthma, child becomes blue in the face.
- Whooping cough with nosebleed.
- Asthma with travel sickness.
- **Ipecac is an important asthma emergency remedy.**

Kali bich. (*kali bichromium*)
- Asthma brought on by change to hot weather.
- Asthma with hard cough and thick tenacious or stringy mucus.
- Snuffles of children, especially fat, chubby babies.
- Inability to breathe through nose. Violent sneezing.
- Profuse watery nasal discharge.
- Thick, green nasal discharge in children.
- **An important remedy for catarrh preceeding asthma.**

Mixed grasses
- A remedy for allergic rhinitis and allergic asthma or hay asthma.
- Asthma brought on during harvesting or grass cutting.

Mixed pollens
- A remedy for allergic rhinitis, allergic asthma and hay fever.
- Asthma which is worse during summer. Asthma from smelling flowers.

Nat. mur. (*natrum muriaticum*)
- Hates sympathy, fuss and company.
- Irritable, weepy. Cries with laughter.
- Always falling in love with the wrong person.
- Common cold. Tendency to frequent recurring colds.
- Asthma or shortness of breath on going up stairs.
- Asthma worse by the sea.
- Dry hair. Ridged nails. Craving for salt.

Nux vom. (poison nut)
- Suits rather thin people, quick, active, nervous, irritable.
- Asthma following the effects of over-indulgence of stimulants such as coffee, tea, alcohol.
- Acid rising. Much stomach pain. Woken at night with indigestion.
- Asthma with fullness in stomach, worse in the morning or after eating.
- Asthma with shallow breathing, very tight chest.
- Asthma with tight, dry hacking cough, sometimes with bloody saliva.

Phosphorus
- Craves company, and touch. Loves being massaged.
- Suits tall, slender, delicate people, with soft dark hair.
- Anxious, restless, can't stand or sit still.
- Asthma, worse in the dark, or before thunderstorms.
- Asthma, worse from cold and cold weather, always better when kept warm.
- Voice rough, husky, can hardly speak above a whisper.
- Cough from constant tickling in throat.
- Chronic asthma spasm. Can hardly walk for difficult breathing.
- Asthma with tendency to lie only on right side. Excessive exhaustion.
- Asthma or cough always worse when going from warm to cold room.

Pulsatilla
- Fair hair and blue eyes, asthma always better in the open air.
- Easily moved to laughter or tears.
- Asthma which cannot breathe in a warm room, must have windows open.
- Cannot tolerate rich foods, greasy foods, cakes, pastries.
- Asthma with thick tenacious catarrh, loss of sense of smell. Cannot breathe through nose at night.

Sepia
This is a remarkable asthma remedy which is best prescribed on the mental symptoms:
- Irritable, indifferent towards loved ones. Apathetic towards work.
- Has lost all ambition. Doesn't want to do anything, work or play.
- Asthma has reduced the sufferer almost to a zombie.
- Asthma with postnatal depression following birth.

Silica
- Fear of failure. Asthma from tension and fears.
- No mental or physical stamina. Asthma from being bullied or threatened. Difficult children. Fidgety, cannot sit still.

- Bad skin at puberty. Long history of recurring chest complaints which have culminated in chronic asthma.
- White flecks in finger nails. Greasy hair. Head sweats.
- Sweaty feet with strong smell.

Sulphur
- Thin, untidy people. Lank hair, strong perspiration smell.
- Always look unwashed even though just bathed.
- Asthma which see-saws with eczema.
- Always hungry, particularly at around 11 a.m. Much offensive wind.
- Asthmatic child always has dirty nose, sore nostrils.
- Asthmatic babies, always hot, kick off bedclothes, feet smell.
- Much offensive wind, sometimes with sulphurous smell.
- Asthma with nappy rash, red irritation around anus.

Symphoricarpus racemosa (snowberry)
- Recommended for persistent vomiting during pregnancy.
- Morning sickness.

Asthmatic's emergency kit
- Aconite for asthma after getting cold.
- Belladonna for asthma and teething.
- Carbo Veg. for elderly asthmatics.
- Ipecac for severe asthma spasms.

Note: When requesting a homoeopathic prescription for a baby ask your pharmacy to prepare the remedy in powder form, or a potentized liquid form which can be dissolved in a little boiled water and given in a feeding bottle. If only pills or pilules are available these can be crushed and dissolved.

7
Vitamins, minerals and trace elements
What are vitamins?

The name vitamin is a general term for a number of unrelated organic substances that occur in many foods. Science has so far identified a large number of these and given each one a letter, and sometimes also a number as in the case of the 'B' group. Doubtless there are more vitamins and minerals yet to be discovered, but at the present time we are aware that of those we know, some can play an important part in the treatment and prevention of asthma.

Vitamins are essential for health, and yet with a few exceptions our bodies cannot manufacture them. We know they are found in very small quantities in all organic foods and most people obtain sufficient quantities of vitamins providing their diet embraces a wide variety of the correct foods. However when a disease condition prevails within the body over a long period of time, a depletion of the body's vital resources slowly takes place. This can produce a lack of certain vital vitamins and minerals which in turn will allow the disease condition to gain control. In order to lay the foundation for a systematic attack on the disease it is wise to make up this depletion, so the vital force of the body is strengthened. This enables the body to assist in treating the disease and gives whatever other treatment being used a greater opportunity for cure. Although asthma is not a disease in the accepted sense of the term, it is a condition which can slowly lower the general health, and should be treated as seriously as a disease. The supplement must be chosen carefully to ensure that the specific needs of the patient are met. For instance, in nervous asthma, the supplement would contain vitamins and minerals valuable for the nervous system, whilst the supplement for the intrinsic asthma sufferer would be designed to strengthen the immune system against recurring infection. Sometimes a simple change in diet is all that is needed to supply the missing vitamin or mineral, and this will be discussed in the next chapter. To ascertain what is needed in the supplement can often be decided by studying the diet of the individual. If the diet has been particularly poor and lacking in the essential elements then a supplement alongside the change in diet would be advised. To arrive at an assessment of mineral or vitamin needs for the average person, you start by comparing the range of food that is regularly eaten with the table of vitamin and mineral values in the following chapter. By observing what foods are regularly omitted from the diet, a fair assessment can be arrived at regarding the vitamins and/or minerals that are most likely to be lacking. In a large number of cases, especially regarding children, faults in the diet are a recurring factor in the underlying cause of the asthma.

Some patients show clear indications of deficiency, in which case dietary advice can be given and the necessary supplement prescribed without hesitation. However there are times when deficiencies show in people who are very careful with their diet: in these cases a faulty metabolism or a deficiency in the food itself must be suspected.

Metabolism

The word metabolism, which comes from a word meaning to change or alter, comprises within itself two other words, *anabolism* and *catabolism*. Metabolism is the sum of all the physical and chemical processes in the body, anabolism is that by which living organized substance is produced and maintained, and catabolism is the transformation by which energy is made available for the uses of the body.

It is important to know that these processes can only take place with the aid of vitamins, and that a deficiency in just one vitamin can upset the whole body.

Vitamins help to regulate our metabolism, which in turn keeps us feeling fit and energetic.

Where do we get our vitamins from?

Vitamins occur in all organic material. That means vegetables, fruit, eggs, meat and fish. Some foods are richer in particular vitamins than others, and the reader is referred to the chapter on diet (Chapter 8) for further information.

Only three vitamins are manufactured by our body: they are D, K_1, and K_2.

Vitamin D is manufactured by the action of sunlight (ultra-violet rays) on the oils of our skin. The manufacturing stops when we develop a suntan.

Vitamin K_1 and K_2 can be formed by natural bacteria in our intestines.

How do we become deficient?

There are a number of ideas regarding this question, among which are poor soil in which the food is grown, manufacturing techniques which deprive the food of essential elements, and environmental poisons such as heavy metals, nitrates, etc which interfere with absorption or destroy them at source.

Many of the people who live in large cities survive without fresh air, sunlight, or good wholesome food, whilst at the same time absorbing large amounts of carbon monoxide and lead from exhaust fumes. Any one of these factors could be contributory to a deficiency which in turn could be responsible for undermining their general health.

Stress is also thought to be a factor which can inhibit the proper digestion of our food, by causing acid in the stomach which subsequently means that we do not get the maximum benefit from each meal. The regular use of medicinal drugs, often the lifeline of an asthmatic, may prove to upset digestion or in themselves cause certain deficiencies.

Processed food

It has been said for many years by alternative medicine that white flour and white sugar and the products that are made from them have undermined the health of the western world. This is due in some measure to the processing through which they are passed depleting their natural nutrients. This processing or bleaching is carried out because the public have been led to prefer 'white' in the mistaken belief that it means pure. When bread is made from totally natural flour it is very dark and coarse-looking, and contains much natural fibre as well as natural vitamins and minerals. The manufacturers and retailers, on the other hand, with the use of high-powered advertising, would have you believe that the goodness taken out by their processing has been replaced and that you are now eating a product that is brimming over with all the essential vitamins and minerals needed for a healthy body.

Many of the nutrients removed during the processing of flour to make it white cannot be replaced; instead the manufacturer replaces a proportion of some of the vitamins and minerals. This makes the advertising misleading to say the least, and the product of questionable taste and quality compared with its wholemeal counterpart. The same argument can be levelled at the processors of sugar and a number of other products on the food markets.

Deficiency through diet

You will also run the risk of vitamin deficiency if you eat only a limited range of foods. I know some children who will not eat any fruit, and will only eat chipped potatoes and baked beans, their favourite meat being beefburgers or sausages.

Some elderly people on a limited budget mistakenly restrict their food intake in favour of heating fuel, without realizing that the restricted diet or poor quality food is undermining their health. This often means they feel the cold more easily and consequently use more heating fuel to keep warm, whereas a healthy diet would provide fuel and energy, which in turn would provide inner heat for their body.

I also know a number of very busy executive types who regularly see clients over a 'business lunch', which means extended lunch hours, often with alcohol. This, plus the stress of talking business over a meal, inevitably leads to an acid stomach which in turn leads to a restriction in the number of different foods that can be consumed without causing distress.

Nutrient utilization and deficiency

There are six main nutrients essential for your health: carbohydrates, proteins, fats, minerals, vitamins, and water. The body utilizes these through its digestive system, but as previously mentioned, if you have a long-term digestive problem it can cause a fault in the assimilation and distribution of one or more of these important factors. Equally, by restricting the range of foods that you eat you reduce the chances of your body obtaining sufficient of each of these factors for the maintenance of its health.

Asthma drugs and vitamin deficiency

It is thought by some authorities that corticosteroids such as cortisone and prednisone can cause a deficiency of vitamins B_6, D, and C.

Important vitamins for asthma

Just as the different types of asthma need different vitamin or mineral supplements, so do the needs of the different age groups vary. A young child with intrinsic asthma would need to be treated entirely differently to a pensioner with extrinsic asthma. Many writers and practitioners over the years have claimed to have discovered the perfect asthmatic diet, but this will never be because of the variable needs of the individual, and the different types of asthma that exist. Likewise, many people have in the past tried a certain vitamin or mineral because it appeared to work wonders for a friend, and then complained bitterly when it failed to work for them. If you experiment in this way you will almost certainly end up being unfairly disillusioned with natural therapies and may miss for ever the opportunity of producing an improvement in your condition. However, there are a small range of vitamins that are commonly used in the treatment of asthma and these are: **A**, **C**, **D** and **E**. Although these vitamins may help some asthma conditions, it is important that the entire range of vitamins and minerals is understood in order to treat the person, and not just the asthma.

- **Vitamins should not be used as a general tonic to improve well-being or as a substitute for bad diet.**

Vitamins and their uses

Vitamins have been found to have a number of important actions on the body's systems or functions. Many are involved in the activity of enzymes, which are substances that promote biochemical reactions in the body.

Below is a brief guide to the areas of the body and the related necessary vitamins:

- **Brain and nervous system:** Folic acid; pantothenic acid (B_5); pyridoxine (B_6); thiamine (B_1); B_{12}; C.
- **Blood vessels:** Vitamin E.
- **Lungs:** Vitamins A and E.
- **Skin:** Niacin (B_3); pyridoxine (B_6); riboflavin (B_2); A; E.
- **Digestion:** Pantothenic acid (B_5); pyridoxine (B_6).
- **Metabolism:** Biotin; folic acid; niacin (B_3); pantothenic acid (B_5); pyridoxine (B_6); riboflavin (B_2); thiamine (B_1); B_{12}; E.
- **Growth:** Folic acid; A; B_{12}.
- **Immune system:** Vitamin C.
- **Blood:** Folic acid; pantothenic acid (B_5); pyridoxine (B_6); B_{12}; E; K.

Recommended daily amounts (RDA)

Guidelines for assessing the nutritional value of diets are called Recommended Daily Amounts. The basis for an RDA is the minimum daily requirement necessary to treat deficiencies of minerals or vitamins.

For each vitamin or mineral listed a suggested RDA is given. If this is not known, then a suggested average daily dose is given. In every case this is meant as the suggested dose in the case of a deficiency and *not* an automatic daily supplement for every reader.

The following abbreviations are used for measurement of dosage:

microgrames=mcg. Milligrames=mg. Grams=g.
International Units=iu.

Vitamin 'A'

This is a fat-soluble vitamin and it can be stored in the body; because of this there is a slight risk of toxicity. The toxic level is considered to be ten times the average daily dose, and then only if taken as more than 100 000 iu daily for many weeks. The toxic dose for infants is above 18 500 iu daily.

- Symptoms of toxicity: hair loss; nausea, vomiting; diarrhoea; dry skin; blurred vision; rashes; bone pains; tiredness; headaches.

If these are experienced the supplement should be stopped.

Benefits for asthmatics

- *Builds resistance to respiratory infections.*
- *Shortens the duration of diseases.*
- Promotes strong bones, *healthy skin*, hair and teeth.
- *Helps in the treatment of Emphysema.*
- Helps weak eyesight and night blindness.

I have seen cases of chronic asthma/eczema show remarkable improvement with regular doses of vitamin A.

- Average daily adult dose=10 000 iu.
- Average daily children's dose=5000 iu.

The 'B' vitamins

Most B vitamins have no direct beneficial effect on the respiratory system, but they are extremely valuable for the nervous system, and in this way their action is used for the effects of asthma as well as 'nervous' or 'stress asthma'. We also know that prolonged illness such as asthma or bronchitis causes a 'run down' feeling, which can often be helped by taking a vitamin B supplement alongside other useful vitamins.

B vitamins are always stronger together, as they act as synergists to each other. This is the reason that most manufacturers produce a B complex supplement. When choosing a multivitamin or B complex supplement, it is wise to check the amount of each B vitamin that it contains, as some manufacturers supply supplement doses too small to be effective. The following list of B vitamins gives the suggested maximum and minimum doses for each; when choosing a multi B supplement choose one that appears to give an average strength somewhere between the maximum and minimum suggestions. Also, in a multi B vitamin complex supplement, B_1 B_2 and B_6 should be in equal strength to each other. As most B vitamins are excreted through the urine, very little is stored in the body; therefore a daily supplement is quite safe to take if you follow the recommended dosages.

In some cases a B complex supplement will cause your urine to turn a darker yellow; this is quite normal and harmless, and indicates that the body is eliminating any excess of vitamin B_2 (riboflavin) which it does not require.

Vitamin B_1 (thiamine). Low potency dose 50mg. High potency dose between 100 and 300mg daily.

Vitamin B_2 (riboflavin). Average daily dose 100 to 300mg.

Vitamin B_3 (niacin=nicotinic acid). Average daily dose 50 to 100mg.

Vitamin B_5 (calcium pantothenate or pantothenic acid). This is useful for countering the effects of prolonged courses of antibiotics. Average daily dose 10 to 100mg.

Vitamin B_6 (pyridoxine). Average daily dose 100 to 300mg.

Vitamin B_{12} (cobalamin). Average daily dose 3mcg. This is the only vitamin that also contains essential minerals. Should be combined with calcium to aid absorption.

Vitamin B_{15} (pangamic acid). Average dose 50 to 100mg. (Not a recognized vitamin, but is known to relieve symptoms of asthma.)

Choline. This is also a member of the B-complex group and is found in combination with B vitamins, it works in harmony with inositol, another member of the B group, and helps to prevent eczema. No RDA has been established. Average daily dose for both choline and inositol is 50 to 500mg.

Folic acid. Another member of the B complex which is

needed if you are a heavy drinker, or if you are taking
more than 2 or 3g of vitamin C daily. It should also be
considered if you are taking any of the following:
aspirin; oestrogens; sulphonamides; phenobarbital.
RDA for adults is 400mcg. For pregnant and lactating
women the RDA is 800mcg.

Para-aminobenzoic acid. A fairly new part of the B-
complex group, a lack of this vitamin can cause eczema.
It is also known to protect against ageing. No RDA
established. Average daily dose 30 to 100mg.

Vitamin C

This vitamin is water soluble and helps in the formation
of collagen, which in turn is important for the repair and
growth of particular cells. This is one of the most popular
vitamins to take as a supplement, as by its action it helps
to oxygenate the blood, which in turn promotes and
accelerates the healing processes. It also acts as a natural
laxative, whilst another important function is its choles-
terol-reducing abilities.

Benefits for asthmatics

An important vitamin for maintaining good health, essential for babies and young children, and particularly for
those asthmatics with long histories of chest infection.

- *Helps in preventing viral and bacterial infections.*
- *Reduces the effects of many allergy-producing substances.*
- *Used in the treatment of, and to prevent, the common cold.*

It is available in syrups, effervescent tablets, and
powder form. Doses vary between 50mg and 10g. The
most popular form is in 1g effervescent tablets which have
an orange or lemon flavour or in syrups which suit young
children and babies.

The best quality vitamin C is that which comes from
rose hips. These contain bioflavonoids as well as other
enzymes that assist the body to digest vitamin C.

The average daily requirement is around 3 grams, but
because the body excretes vitamin C within two to three
hours, it is best taken 1g three times daily, or in a time-
release capsule. Carbon monoxide destroys vitamin C,
and so people living in densely populated environments

such as cities should seriously consider a daily supplement. Pregnant women, particularly if they suffer from asthma, and women taking the birth control pill also need more vitamin C.

- Babies with asthma: 50mg twice daily as rose hip syrup.
- Average daily dose adults and children: 1 to 3g. Mega doses=5 to 15g.

Beware of any liquid vitamin C preparation which contains artificial additives.

Vitamin D

This is one of the few vitamins which the body is able to manufacture for itself. It does this by the action of sunlight (ultra-violet) on the skin. In the treatment of asthma I have experienced some marked results with the use of ultra-violet treatment. Asthma sufferers who live in cities, or work indoors away from sunlight, children or old people with asthma or bronchitis, and those who suffer recurring colds should be taking a supplement of this vitamin.

Benefits for asthmatics
No direct benefit to the lungs, but its beneficial action on skin complaints, such as eczema which is often associated with asthma, improves the underlying cause of the asthma in some cases. For the intrinsic asthmatic this vitamin is important as it helps maintain resistance to disease. It helps the body to assimilate calcium and phosphorus, as well as vitamin A. In combination with vitamins A and C it is valuable as a cold prevention treatment.

- RDA for adults: 400 iu.

It is recommended that a dose of over 5 000 iu per day should be avoided.

Vitamin E

This is a fat-soluble vitamin which is composed of a number of compounds known as tocopherols. It works in harmony with vitamin A, and selenium which enhance its action.

Like vitamins B and C it is not stored in the body, and between 60 and 70 per cent of daily intake is excreted.

It helps to supply oxygen to the body, retards cellular ageing, is a diuretic and can lower blood pressure.

Benefits for asthmatics

- Asthmatic women who are pregnant, lactating, or who take the birth pill, need more vitamin E.
- Asthmatic women who are experiencing the menopause should increase their intake of this vitamin.
- Asthmatics who drink chlorinated water are also advised to increase their intake of E.

As an ointment or cream it is absorbed through the skin, and is a useful ointment for eczema.

Essentially non-toxic, the average recommended daily dose is between 200 iu, and 2000 iu.

You will increase your need for vitamin A if you are taking vitamin E.

Vitamin K

There are three K vitamins: K_1 K_2 and K_3. The first two can be manufactured by natural bacteria in the intestine. Sometimes a deficiency may cause coeliac disease, but this is rare, as we take sufficient of this vitamin naturally from a number of different foods. Because of this, it is not often found in vitamin supplement capsules.

Average daily dose 300mcg.

No RDA established.

Doses above 500mcg are not recommended.

Vitamin P

Citrin plus rutin and hesperidin form vitamin P.

It is often found in vitamin C complex tablets as it works in harmony with vitamin C.

Benefits for asthmatics

- For the intrinsic asthmatic it helps to build resistance against infection.
- It is valuable for conditions which are caused by capillary fragility (weakening of small arteries), and some cases of high blood pressure are helped by this vitamin, as well as varicose veins.

Average adult dose is 100mg.

How important are minerals?

Minerals are vital to our health in numerous ways, as without minerals present in the body vitamins cannot be absorbed or do their work. This is one of the reasons that most manufacturers produce vitamins and minerals together in one supplement.

For the average person the world of minerals can be even more confusing than the world of vitamins. It is hoped the following guide will enable you to decide your individual needs. We know that minerals are essential for our health; unfortunately some people mistakenly believe that the more you take, the healthier you become. However, it is well to remember that too much of one mineral can deplete us of others, whilst the absence of one can prevent the absorption of others.

There are no doubt more discoveries for medical science yet to make, both in the number of minerals present in the body, and in their role in the maintenance of health.

We do know that the important active minerals so far discovered in the body are: calcium; chlorine; chromium; cobalt; copper; fluorine; iodine; iron; magnesium; manganese; molybdenum; phosphorus; potassium; selenium; sodium; vanadium; zinc.

Of these there are six that are more important to our health and of which the necessary daily intake is known. These are: calcium; iodine; iron; magnesium; phosphorus; zinc.

Calcium

There is more calcium in our body than any other mineral, and most of it is found in our bones and teeth.

Calcium and phosphorus together are needed for healthy bones and teeth, whilst calcium needs vitamin D to help its absorption into the body.

For women calcium and iron are the two most commonly deficient minerals, and calcium helps to metabolize iron.

There has been much discussion regarding the condition of osteoporosis (weakening of bone strength), and the lack of calcium due to the menopause in women. There is no evidence so far to support the claim that taking increased calcium will prevent this condition. Indeed in some areas where the water is very chalky, increasing the calcium intake may lead to the formation of kidney or gall stones.

- RDA: 800 to 1200mg daily.

Iodine

Iodine is needed for thyroid activity. It influences the thyroid gland, which in turn controls metabolism. A lack of this mineral can undermine thyroid activity, which can slow you down mentally and physically as well as causing weight increase.

- RDA: 80 to 150mcg. (A general guide to dosage is 1mcg per kilo body weight.)
- For asthma sufferers who are pregnant or breastfeeding the RDA is 125 to 150mcg.

Iron

This is an essential mineral for life, as it plays a part in the production of red blood corpuscles. The body only assimilates approximately 10 per cent of iron intake. To help in the assimilation of iron the body needs copper, cobalt, manganese and vitamin C.

Your body will need more iron if you drink large quantities of tea or coffee. Women lose twice as much iron each month as men.

Some types of iron supplement (ferrous sulphate) can cause constipation; the best type of iron supplement is hydrolysed-protein chelate which is kind to the system.

Iron supplements should not be given to children without a doctor's advice.

- RDA: 10 to 18mg.

Magnesium

Magnesium plays an important part in metabolism. Without it the body cannot absorb vitamin C, calcium, phosphorus, sodium or potassium. Calcium and magnesium are found in perfect balance in the mineral dolomite: the balance should always be twice as much calcium as magnesium.

Magnesium can help to prevent heart attacks, calcium deposits, as well as kidney and gallstones.

People living in a hard water area rarely need a magnesium supplement.
- RDA: 300 to 400mg. (Large amounts can be toxic if your calcium and phosphorus intakes are high.)

Phosphorus

This mineral is present in every cell in the body and is essential for health. For phosphorus to do its work properly it needs calcium and vitamin D. If you have too much iron, aluminium or magnesium in the body it will interfere with the work that phosphorus must do.

On the other hand, too much phosphorus in the body will upset the mineral balance and cause a decrease in the calcium levels. Because our diets are usually high in phosphorus, calcium deficiencies are common.
- RDA for adults: 800 to 1200mg.

Zinc

An important mineral in many respects, zinc is responsible for the maintenance of enzyme systems and cells. It is essential for protein synthesis and the formation of insulin.

It maintains the acid/alkaline balance of the body as well as the stability of the blood. It is now believed to play an important part in brain function and is being linked with the treatment for schizophrenia and Alzheimer's disease (senile dementia).

Excessive sweating can cause a loss of up to 3mg of zinc per day. A high calcium and/or iron level is thought to cause zinc deficiency as well as a high fibre diet and the long-term use of laxatives. Most zinc in foods is lost through processing, or is lacking because of soil that is poor in nutrients. If you are considering a zinc supplement, you will also need more vitamin A.

A liquid form of zinc is now available, which is suitable for babies and children.
- RDA for adults: 15 to 20mg.
- Pregnant or lactating women: 25mg.

Professor D. Bryce-Smith, Professor of Organic Chemistry at Reading University, has written a paper on the 'Diagnosis of Zinc Deficiency' in which he explores the symptoms and causes of zinc deficiency and also explains a simple taste test to determine zinc deficiency. It is especially useful in diagnosing children, and copies of the paper are available from: Felmore Ltd Health Publications, 1 Lambert Road, P.O. Box 1, Tunbridge Wells, TN2 3EQ.

What are chelated minerals?

Chelated, (pronounced *keylated*), refers to a process which is used to change minerals into a more easily digestible form for our body to absorb.

Chelated minerals are a little more expensive to buy, but worth considering: you run the risk of taking unchelated minerals for months before finding out that you have not been absorbing them as you should.

Choosing a supplement

Always buy a good quality supplement, preferably one that has been recommended by your practitioner, or go to a well-established health food store and ask advice.

If you suffer from extrinsic asthma you should check that the coating and contents do not contain artificial colourants. You can purchase special hypo-allergic formulae.

You should also check the quantities of each ingredient, which will be printed on the label to see that they fall within the suggested dietary daily need.

The following are examples of well-balanced supplements:

Vitamin B complex (Medium strength)
- Vitamin B_1: 50mg.
- Vitamin B_2: 50mg.
- Vitamin B_{12}: 50mg.
- Nicotinamide (B_3): 50mg.
- Folic acid: 400mcg.
- Pantothenic acid (B_5): 50mg.
- Biotin: 50mcg.
- Choline: 50mg.
- Inositol: 50mg.
- PABA: 50mg.

A high potency B complex would contain each of the above ingredients at double strength.

Multi mineral/vitamin supplement (1 capsule per day)
- Vitamin A: 7500 iu.
- Vitamin D: 400 iu.
- Vitamin C: 250mg.
- Vitamin E: 150 iu.
- Vitamin B_1: 75mg.
- Vitamin B_2: 75mg.
- Vitamin B_6: 75mg.
- Vitamin B_{12}: 75mcg.

108   *The Asthma Action Plan*

- Nicotinamide: 75mg.
- PABA: 75mg.
- Vitamin B_5: 75mg.
- Biotin: 75mcg.
- Folic acid: 400mcg.
- Magnesium chelate: 1.5mg.
- Manganese: 0.6mg.
- Choline: 75mg.
- Inositol: 75mg.
- Rutin: 25mg.
- Bioflavonoids: 25mg.
- Hesperidin complex: 6mg.
- Iodine: 0.15mg.
- Calcium: 10mg.
- Potassium: 1mg.
- Iron: 1mg.
- Zinc: 1.5mg.
- Copper: 25mcg.
- Selenium: 25mcg.

A balanced formula for children (chewable tablets)
- Vitamin A: 4000 iu.
- Vitamin D: 400 iu.
- Vitamin C: 60mg.
- Vitamin B_1: 2mg.
- Vitamin B_2: 2.4mg.
- Vitamin B_6: 2mg.
- Vitamin B_{12}: 10mcg.
- Vitamin E: 3.4 iu.
- Biotin: 10mcg.
- Calcium pantothenate: 2mg.
- Calcium: 19mg.
- Copper: 0.2mg.
- Iron: 12mg.
- Magnesium: 22mg.
- Choline: 2mg.
- Potassium: 4mg.
- Inositol: 2mg.
- Nicotinamide: 10mg.

Trace elements

The twelve biochemic remedies

These are known as mineral salts and were shown to be important to health by Dr Schuessler in 1873 when he published the first of numerous papers on the subject of the results of molecular disturbance, and the subsequent cure by the administration of a specific cell salt.

These he isolated into twelve of what he considered to be the most important to the body. The whole number of tissue salts together constitute only 5 per cent of the minerals in the body, and yet they play a vital part.

The five principals of Dr Schuessler's Biochemistry are:

1. Disease does not occur if cell metabolism is normal.
2. Cell metabolism is in turn normal if cell nutrition is adequate.

3. Nutritional substances are either of an organic or inorganic nature where the body is concerned.
4. The ability of the cells to assimilate, utilize and excrete is impaired if there is a deficiency in the mineral (tissue salt) constituent of cellular tissues.
5. Adequate cell nutrition may be restored and cellular metabolism normalized by supplying the required mineral salts to the organism in finely divided assimilable form.

The tissue salts are inorganic matter and were proved by Dr Schuessler in the homoeopathic dilution of 6x to render them into an assimilable form so that the body could use them more easily. The logical reasoning was that if the body lacked a certain amount of a particular salt it was due either to the body's inability to absorb it from its food (metabolism), or that it was deficient in the food. Either way, the 6x dilution of the salt helped by enabling the body to accept it more easily if metabolism was at fault, and also acting as a supplement if the diet was deficient. By treating a deficiency of these tissue salts you are in fact looking below the surface symptoms and seeking to treat the cause of your asthma. In some cases this revolves around the body's inability to overcome recurring infections thereby producing fertile ground for the appearance of intrinsic asthma; in other cases a deficiency of a tissue salt may upset the delicate balance within the body which in turn may make it extremely sensitive to certain allergens.

To ascertain which tissue salt you should consider as a treatment for your asthma, other symptoms which are present should also be considered; the following brief description of the twelve tissue salts seeks to guide the asthmatic in choosing the correct one.

A guide to the leading symptoms of deficiency

Calcarea fluor
Necessary for the elasticity of the skin, muscular tissue and blood vessels, and for the surface of the bones and the enamel of teeth.
- **Symptoms of deficiency:** frequent cold sores; eczema; hardened glands; swollen veins or arteries; small joints swollen.

Calc. Fluor is often indicated in chronic bronchitic conditions and intrinsic asthma. It would be indicated for intrinsic asthma if any of the previous symptoms are present as well.

Calcarea phos.
This mineral is necessary for the building of strong bones and teeth, which makes it a particularly important remedy for children. It also acts on the blood, helping in the formation of blood corpuscles, as well as gastric juices. In this role it becomes an important trace element to assist in faulty metabolism.
- **Symptoms of deficiency:** Teething problems in babies, e.g. teeth develop too slowly and decay rapidly; poor circulation; bones brittle, fractures do not heal; itching skin in old people; rheumatism worse from weather changes; acid stomach; children lacking concentration.

This tissue salt is for young and old alike and strongly indicated for intrinsic asthma when one or more of the above symptoms are present.

Calcarea sulph.
This trace element plays an important part in the health of the skin cells: it prevents cell disintegration. A deficiency of this salt promotes undue suppuration from conditions such as boils, abscesses and ulcers. It is also indicated in such conditions as varicose ulcers which refuse to heal, and boils which have a thick, yellow pus or matter. It is particularly indicated for that most troublesome of teenage conditions, acne.
- **Symptoms of deficiency:** any skin condition that is slow to heal; pimples; spots; boils, etc; loss of hair with dandruff; symptoms that are worse from working in water or getting wet.

The remedy to be considered for both intrinsic or extrinsic asthma when the skin is also involved and showing these particular symptoms.

Ferrum phos.
Iron plays an essential part in forming haemoglobin which carries oxygen to every part of the body. It provides strength to the blood vessels, and is the leading tissue salt

to be thought of in all inflammatory conditions. It is the most frequently needed of the tissue salts because most diseases commence with inflammation of one kind or another.

- **Symptoms of deficiency:** Headaches in children; nose bleeds; flushed face; commencement of bronchitis with burning soreness; loss of voice, hoarseness; simple anaemia; symptoms arising from high blood pressure.

Again a tissue salt for both young and old, it is especially useful in asthma of children who are tired and debilitated, as well as for many complaints associated with advancing years. It should form at least a part of the treatment where there are recurring infections which lead to intrinsic asthma.

Kali mur.

This mineral salt is found in every tissue of the body except the bones. Its particular role is to unite with albumin to form fibrin. A deficiency of this salt causes a release of albumin which in turn causes the production of a thick, sticky discharge from the mucous membranes in the body. It is an important mineral salt for the asthmatic as in both intrinsic and extrinsic asthma it is the formation of thick sticky mucus which hinders the breathing and causes the frightening wheezing and troublesome night cough. It is indicated where there is a white or grey coating of the tongue, throat or tonsils, in glandular swellings, skin eruptions with white or yellow pus, and in cases where the blood has thickened with a tendency to form clots.

- **Symptoms of deficiency:** sick headaches; discharges from the eyes; catarrh of the middle ear; tinnitus; blocked nose; second stage of all respiratory infections; wheezing, rattling congestion; croup; eczema; warts; chilblains; shingles.

Kali phos.

This tissue salt is the great nerve nutrient, but is present throughout the body and performs an antiseptic action on the tissues. It is strongly indicated in all conditions which have been produced or aggravated by nervous exhaustion or continual emotional strain. This makes it a prime treatment for nervous asthma regardless of its intrinsic or extrinsic foundation. A deficiency produces melancholia, irritability, fearfulness, timidity and general prostration. Its symptoms are aggravated by noise, by physical or mental exertion, and movement after rest.

• **Symptoms of deficiency:** anxiety; poor memory; sleeplessness; shyness, excessive blushing; nervous headaches; neuralgia; nervous or hay asthma; palpitations from exertion; nervous skin diseases; shingles.

A strongly indicated treatment for any asthma which is aggravated by any of the above symptoms.

Kali sulph.

This tissue salt is responsible for carrying oxygen to the skin and works in harmony with Ferr Phos. A deficiency causes a lack of oxygen to the skin and this can produce symptoms of chilliness, and inflammations which move from place to place. It can also produce a desire for fresh, cool air. It promotes perspiration and is therefore invaluable in skin conditions which are dry, scaly or crusty. All symptoms are aggravated in a warm room and towards evening, always better in the cool, fresh air.

• **Symptoms of deficiency:** headaches from stuffy atmospheres; dandruff and hair loss; catarrhal deafness with inflammation of the ear; colds with slimy yellow mucus; colic pain; chronic stomach wind with sulphurous gas; skin, hot, dry and harsh; nail diseases.

Magnesia phos.

This mineral salt acts as an antispasmodic of the delicate white nerve fibres of both nerve and muscle; it unites with water and albumin to nourish these fibres. A deficiency causes cramps, sharp darting pains, or neuralgia. It suits thin, lean, emaciated people who are highly nervous.

In view of its beneficial action on spasmodic conditions it is to be particularly considered in certain asthmatic conditions.

• **Symptoms of deficiency:** headaches, darting or stabbing relieved by warm applications; partial vision, half vision; migraine with sparks before eyes; facial neuralgia; teeth sensitive to cold; craving for sugar; aversion to acids or coffee; spasms or cramps of the stomach; trembling of hands; twitching over the body; cramp.

Natrum mur.

Sodium chloride is familiar to everyone as salt, it is a constituent of every part of the body, both liquid and solid. We are 70 per cent water, and without this vital mineral salt we just could not survive. It helps to control the fluid balance in the body, and a deficiency causes a watery and bloated appearance, the person becomes languid and drowsy. It also controls the amount of water in the blood as well as certain digestive acids. A deficiency is sometimes indicated when there is a salt craving accompanied with runny colds and thirst, a dry constipation, hangnails, and cold sores are also among its leading deficiency symptoms. Its overproduction of mucus symptoms make it an important tissue salt in the treatment of some asthma symptoms.

- **Symptoms of deficiency:** hammering headaches; depression; drowsy, tired; violent thirst; acid stomach with ravenous hunger; aversion to bread; cracked lips; runny colds with clear mucus; excessive sneezing; greasy skin; soreness in bends of knees or elbows; itching along margin of scalp; eczema of eyebrows or behind ears.

An important mineral salt, as without it other salts sometimes cannot work, its symptoms are worse in the morning, during cold weather and especially by the sea.

Natrum phos.

This mineral salt is present throughout the body and in nerve and brain cells. It has a particular action in splitting lactic acid into carbonoic acid and water; it forms an important trio with Nat Mur. and Nat Sulph., and between them they control the body fluids. This can be extremely important in some forms of asthma, particularly the type of asthma which is affected by changes in the weather. The action of this tissue salt is indicated wherever there is a dyspeptic condition arising from fatty or greasy foods, particularly babies who get stomach upsets from milk and sugar feeds.

All discharges are a creamy golden yellow, from the eyes as well as the mouth. During pregnancy a deficiency can be indicated by morning sickness accompanied by vomiting of sour fluids.

- **Symptoms of deficiency:** headache on crown of head; migraine with intense pressure and nausea; eyelids glued together upon waking; acid or coppery taste in mouth; grinding of teeth at night; heartburn; pain two hours after eating.

Symptoms can be aggravated in the afternoon and evening and from fresh air.

Natrum sulph.

The action of this salt is to regulate the intercellular fluids by controlling the amount of fluid in the tissues and the blood. It helps to control bile and also to eliminate excess water from the system. A deficiency of this important mineral salt causes an imbalance of fluids which can cause the individual to act like a human barometer. In certain asthma sufferers their symptoms would be definitely aggravated in damp weather; in fact they may be able to predict a change from dry to wet weather by their asthma symptoms.

- **Symptoms of deficiency:** sensitive scalp, head painful when combed; vertigo with stomach upset; burning around eyelids; green/brown coating of tongue; bitter taste; humid asthma; difficulty breathing in damp weather; jaundice; sandy deposit in urine; diarrhoea; cannot bear tight clothing around waist.

The symptoms of asthma are aggravated by using water in any form, or even eating fish, or plants which are grown in water. Also aggravations are experienced from damp, rainy weather, living in damp buildings, or on low-lying ground or near marshes.

Silicea

This tissue salt was also mentioned in the chapter on homoeopathy, and the guiding symptoms of deficiency are very similar to the homoeopathic provings. Silica is a mineral which is prevalent throughout the body; it is necessary for connective tissue, bones, blood, skin, hair, nails, and mucous membrane. A deficiency will not only undermine the immune system but will also give rise to an over-sensitivity of the mucous membrane. This means that a deficiency would affect both intrinsic as well as extrinsic asthmas: intrinsic asthmatics would experience recurring infections as well as a permanent catarrhal aggravation due to the immune system being lowered and the over-sensitivity of the mucous membranes. The extrinsic asthmatic would also be affected by the over-sensitivity of the mucous membranes to certain allergens, but if a deficiency of this tissue salt was the underlying cause a cure could only be expected if the deficiency was corrected. The action of this mineral is deep and long-lasting; it can slowly undermine the vital force of the body and give rise to a weakened constitution.

- **Symptoms of deficiency:** premature loss of hair; greasy hair; difficulty in concentration; lack of confidence, or determination; head sweats, particularly in children; styes; boils; recurring mouth ulcers; nails brittle and with white flecking; strong smelling and profuse foot sweat; fidgety children; hyperactivity.

In all cases of asthma when a Silicea deficiency is indicated, the deficiency must be corrected before improvement from other medication can be expected.

Using the tissue salts

If more than one tissue salt is indicated by the symptoms it is perfectly safe to take two or three at the same time: they do not clash. If you have a chronic asthma problem it would be advisable to take the indicated remedy or remedies every two or three hours throughout the day over several months, gradually reducing the frequency of the dose until you are taking them just three times daily. The remedy is stopped when all symptoms have gone. Should you need to take more than one tissue salt it is best that they be taken alternately with each other.

If you are treating an acute attack of asthma, it may be advisable to take the indicated remedy every fifteen minutes until relief is experienced, and then reduce the dose to every two hours until all symptoms have gone. Thereafter as a prevention against a return attack you should take a dose before meals.

Further information books:

Thorsons Complete Guide to Vitamins and Minerals, by Leonard Mervyn (Thorsons).
The Vitamin Bible, by Earl Mindell (Arlington Books).

8
Food and asthma

I have deliberately called this chapter 'Food and Asthma' because the word 'diet' to many people conjures up pictures of dull meals, of never being able to eat in restaurants, of feeling hungry, deprived and miserable. To the asthmatic, diet is of great importance and can mean the difference between life in its fullest meaning, or existence.

In this chapter I hope to prove that eating the correct foods is an enjoyable experience, and can benefit both extrinsic and intrinsic asthma symptoms.

In the previous chapter on vitamins and minerals it was explained how vital they are to our health, and that a deficiency of vitamins and/or minerals can often be traced to a wrong way of eating. This is due in part to ignorance which commences in school due to a lack of nutritional education, and in part to a lack of discipline in some people who will only eat the things that appeal to them.

Nutritional education

This should be an essential part of our knowledge because it leads to the maintenance of our energy and vitality, and is contributory to our physical and mental abilities.

Our educational system, in the past, has not included in its curriculum any nutritional or general health education, as a result of which, young people grew up in ignorance of the importance of food factors to their health. They in turn had children who were raised in the same mould; this has now resulted in generations of ignorance regarding the importance of food to our health. This ignorance in turn has allowed a whole range of food products on to the supermarket shelf by public demand.

These include instant meals, potato crisps, confectionery, dried instant snacks re-activated by the addition of hot water, white bread and numerous fruit-flavoured milky drinks and yoghurts, many containing little nutritional value, and others manufactured with brilliant colours and artificial flavourings to appeal to the young mind but containing dubious substances used to colour, add taste, emulsify and preserve.

'E' for danger

Before we begin exploring the foods which you should eat, it would be wise to have some knowledge of the foods or substances which you must avoid because of the potential danger they offer to the asthmatic.

Among the substances which are used by manufacturers for colouring and/or preserving certain foods are some which should be avoided, particularly by asthmatics who also suffer aspirin or skin allergies, especially young babies and children with asthma and/or eczema.

These additives are identified by 'E' numbers, of which there are hundreds used by food manufacturers. The majority of them have been proved absolutely harmless and safe. However, a number of them still in use in the UK have been identified as a cause of asthma aggravation as well as allergic skin and respiratory conditions, and in some cases they have proved to be the cause of behavioural and learning problems in children.

The following list is of those 'E' numbers which have been known to cause a reaction in some asthma conditions, to aspirin allergy sufferers, and in some allergic conditions.

In the UK, government legislation now ensures that the *majority* of foods are labelled with a list of contents including the preservatives and colourants they contain. The asthmatic should carefully check the label on all food and drink substances to ensure that it does not contain any of the following 'E' numbers:

E102	E107	E110	E122	E123	E124	E131
E132	E155	E210	E211	E212	E214	E214
E215	E216	E217	E218	E219	E220	E221
E222	E223	E224	E226	E227	E250	E310
E311	E312	E321				

Food products in which these 'E' numbers may be found

Alcoholic beverages
Beer
Barbecue Sauce
Bacon
Campden tablets
Coloured fizzy drinks
Custard powder
Chewing gum
Crystallized fruit
Cured meat
Breakfast cereal
Fruit juices
Fruit squash and cordials
Flavouring syrups
Gravy granules
Hot chocolate mix
Ice cream
Instant puddings
Jelly
Marzipan
Marmalade
Packet mashed potatoes
Orange jelly biscuits
Pork sausages
Pickled onions
Pickles
Pickled red cabbage
Quick frozen shrimps, prawns, lobsters or chips
Soups [tinned or packet]
Smoked cod
Smoked frankfurters
Scotch eggs
Sweets
Salami
Salad cream and dressing
Snack meals
Table olives
Tinned meat

Trifle mix
Tinned apple sauce
Tinned fruit pie fillings
Fruit yogurt
Yogurt whip
Bottled sauces
Pre-packed beetroot
Packet bacon steaks
Carton salads
Cider
Chicory and coffee essence
Cake mixes
Chocolate cakes
Caviar
Glacé fruit
Cured meat products
Frozen pizza
'Exotic' dried fruits and nuts
Freeze drinks
Fruit pulp and purée
Glycerine lemon and honey products
Dessert topping
Ice lollies
Jam
Lemon curd
Margarines and shortenings
Mustard
Oyster sauce
Orange squash
Concentrated pineapple juice
Packet breadcrumbs
Preserved egg yolk
Pickled cucumbers
Packet cheesecake mix
Swiss roll
Smoked haddock

Salted peanuts
Shells of medicinal
  capsules
Seafood dressing
Soused herring and
  mackerel
Soya sauce
Soup concentrates

Turkey and ham loaf
Tongue
Tinned shrimps and
  prawns
Tinned pears
Wine
Vegetable oil
Yogurt

- **A warning to mothers with young children:** Some
  liquid Vitamin C preparations may contain 'E' numbers.

A number of food manufacturers now produce many
products which do not contain any additives whatsoever.
Nevertheless I believe that the evidence is overwhelm-
ingly in favour of a change in the eating habits of asthma
sufferers, and the following pages contain advice for both
extrinsic and intrinsic asthmatics.

Children and food

The mother with a child that suffers extrinsic asthma may
well be forgiven for throwing up her hands in despair
after reading through the list of potentially dangerous
foods, because it contains many of the foods or sauces
that are used in the average kitchen. It is without doubt
the most difficult era in which to bring up an asthmatic
child on the correct foods, because as the mother is
teaching the child to avoid those foods which may promote an asthma attack, television commercials are beguil-
ing them with the use of high-powered advertising into
believing that the chocolate bars, fizzy drinks, crisps, and
numerous convenience foods, are in fact good for them.

A fact, whether by coincidence or not, is that the
majority of these products which are nationally advertised
contain ingredients which appear on the danger 'E' list for
asthmatics. Their nutritional value is generally poor, and
if taken in quantities in place of regular meals, these goods
will prove generally unhealthy for the child.

A child needs to be trained and encouraged to enjoy
the foods which are good for it, and the training should
begin when the baby is weaned from milk to solid foods.

If you are attempting the management of your asthmatic child's diet for the first time, it is certain to be difficult, but with care and determination an average 'mum' can find acceptable alternatives to the crisps and chocolate bars and find ways of preparing disliked food that will appeal.

Case history of Master X

Master X was 8 years old when he was first brought to see me by his grandmother. He was a very small child with an underdeveloped body and with the typical curved spine and hunched shoulders of the chronic asthma sufferer. Examination revealed a chronic condition of eczema over the entire body, which his grandmother assured me was 'not bad at all lately'.

This was a typical case of intrinsic asthma, even down to the history of tuberculosis on his father's side. Every breath was an effort for Master X, and this together with his thin crooked body, and the grey pallor of his face, produced a very sad picture. He had lost countless days of schooling, and because his mother, who was a single parent, needed to work, Master X spent most of his days with his grandmother or wandering the streets. When questioned on his eating habits, it transpired that Master X was allowed to eat only the things he 'fancied' – 'Poor little mite,' said his grandmother, 'what else can we do? He doesn't have any fun like his friends.' The things he liked turned out to be – yes, you've guessed it – chips, beefburgers, cola, and chocolate biscuits. He had not eaten fresh meat or vegetables since he was two years old, and he hated fruit! His mother was contacted and she readily agreed to co-operate. Master X was given a points score sheet and a food guide sheet which contained all the things he hated. The deal was that he could have one glass of cola and two chocolate biscuits per day, providing he followed the food guide. He was to deduct 10 points for each glass of cola or chocolate biscuit that he ate daily over the allotted amount, but he could add 20 points for each day that he managed to follow the guide. At the end of four weeks his points were to be added up and I promised him £1.00 for every 100 points he had scored, plus £2 for every length of the school swimming pool he could swim after he had been following the food guide for a month.

I examined him a month later and even I was surprised at the change in his skin. Not only was it clear of eczema, but he actually had a colour to his cheeks, his breathing was almost normal, and he had won the maximum points – 560! Both his grandmother and mother assured me he had not cheated once, and this I could certainly believe from his improvement. The story was concluded a week later when, in addition to the £5.60 he originally won from me, I found myself parting with a £20.00 note at the end of a fantastic 10-length swim. It was the best investment I had ever made.

Starting school can present difficulties because once at school the child is often given a choice of meals, and it is natural for the child to opt for the meal which appeals mostly to the taste buds, and ignore the fresh vegetables which he is encouraged to eat at home. I am sure we all know of some children who spend their daily school meal money on potato crisps, beefburgers and chocolate bars and often go for weeks without a proper meal. The parents, unaware of this, will prepare a light meal after school in the mistaken belief that the child has already had a 'square meal' whilst at school.

Should you suspect this situation is developing with your child, a discreet word with someone in authority at school will often ensure that your child is encouraged on your behalf to eat the correct foods.

The good food guide for all types of asthma

To achieve glowing health it is vital that the diet should include a variety of fresh foods, among which should be fresh vegetables and fruit – both raw and cooked – good quality meat, poultry and fish, plus a regular intake of fresh water or fresh fruit juices.

This will not only help to improve the asthma but if eczema is present the skin will also benefit from the change in diet.

The following 'Ten Steps Guide' is a sound way to commence the general changes needed toward a more healthy way of eating. It is based on the Schauss/Schoenthaler Diet which has been used with great success in the USA in helping allergy sensitive and hyperactive children.

Ten steps to food control

1. Replace sweetened breakfast cereals with non-sweetened varieties.
2. Replace sugar on the table with honey.
3. Substitute wholemeal bread in place of white bread.
4. Soft drinks should be replaced with a selection of fruit and vegetable juices.
5. Wash all canned fruits, if packed in syrup, with cold running water before serving.
6. Use brown rice to replace white rice.
7. Processed foods should be replaced with fresh foods.
8. Snack foods which are high in sugar, fat or refined carbohydrates should be replaced by fresh fruit and vegetables, plus nuts, cheeses and wholegrain biscuits.
9. Artificially coloured or flavoured foods should be avoided where possible.
10. Place all fresh meat into a pan of boiling water for 10 minutes, remove, throw away the water, then proceed to cook in the chosen way.

Beginning the changes with children

Children are notoriously difficult when it comes to introducing new foods and tastes, and would often rather not eat than try something different. It is wise to begin the changes in subtle ways, for instance by changing the usual orange squash in the cupboard for fresh fruit drinks without additives. Later a little chopped fresh or tinned fruit can be added on top of the breakfast cereal. Not all the foods that children love are bad for them. For instance, many children love baked beans in tomato sauce; beans provide a source of high protein and providing there are no additives, can be given regularly. If the child craves foods such as fish fingers or beefburgers, these too can be given providing they are not frozen, and are prepared from fresh meat or fish.

To encourage a wider variety of foods, commence by serving with their favourite beans and burger, some fresh cooked green cabbage sprinkled with a little vinegar, or cabbage cooked with a chopped onion and tossed in butter.

Baked jacket potatoes, which are rich in vitamins and minerals, and not so fattening as their boiled or roasted counterparts, can be served with a variety of interesting fillings, in place of chips.

Most children hate salads, and who can blame them when you examine the average salad of today which mostly consists of limp lettuce, indifferent cucumber, and tomatoes?

Try preparing a salad by tearing the lettuce into small pieces, slicing the tomatoes into quarters, adding a sliced onion, some thinly sliced raw courgettes (zucchini), small pieces of raw cauliflower florets, sliced raw mushrooms, cubes of wholemeal bread that have been deep-fried, and a sprinkle of sunflower, sesame and pumpkin seeds. Add a little vinegar, one dessertspoon of vegetable or olive oil and one teaspoonful of walnut oil. Toss thoroughly and serve. Most children will eat this type of salad.

With a little time and trouble you can slowly educate a child's palate to appreciate good food, and later in this chapter you will be given further ideas on preparing foods, both raw and cooked, which will appeal to both children and adults.

Beginning the changes with adults

In this modern society the demand and supply of convenience foods has caused a lowering of the standards of quality that at one time were taken for granted. Although we now have methods of temporarily holding food in 'suspension' from fresh, by methods such as quick freezing, preserving with chemicals, and more recently with a technique using radiation, the product when eventually cooked lacks something which its fresh counterpart has.

As we continue to live in larger communities, expanding our housing projects on to agricultural land, and with the world population increasing its demand for food, it becomes increasingly more difficult to avoid buying these instant and convenience foods. Partly as a consequence of this, a large proportion of the population suffer a high acid level in their bodies, which impedes proper digestion, which leads to a higher acid level. Sometimes the long-term taking of an asthma drug will upset the digestion and produce a tendency toward an acid condition.

A return to the proper levels of acid and alkali in our bodies helps produce a marked improvement in energy and health, and is a good point from which to commence a new way of eating for both extrinsic and intrinsic sufferers.

The acid/alkaline balance

It is thought that the acid/alkaline balance in our body should be on a scale of 80 per cent alkaline to 20 per cent acid. However, due in part to dietary factors, such as eating the wrong foods and the addition of preservatives and colourants etc, plus the increasing tendency to drink more alcohol, the majority of people end up with 80 per cent acid and 20 per cent alkaline balance. This can upset our metabolism and lead to a deficiency in vitamins or minerals.

Another factor which causes an acid condition to build in our body is stress. We eat too fast, and we do not take enough exercise between meals. Perhaps we should take a lesson from our European counterparts who look upon mealtimes as a social occasion. They eat in a leisurely manner, often taking time off between courses; care is taken in the choosing and preparation of food, and herbs are widely used to help digestion.

The acid/alkaline diet: a nine-day cleansing programme

The following nine-day cleansing diet will help produce the correct acid/alkaline balance in your body, and give you a marvellous start to your 'new way of eating' programme. It will help to ensure that your body metabolizes to the maximum every mouthful of food that you eat in future, and this in turn will help produce that 'glowing health'.

- **Should you experience any major aggravation to your asthma symptons whilst on this diet it would be wise to stop and seek the advice of your doctor.**

Cleansing: days 1, 2 and 3

Putting yourself on a completely alkaline diet for three days encourages the rapid release of stored waste matter. Your body will rapidly throw off toxins just as it would if you were on a fast, but unlike in fasting, the alkalinity of the fruits helps to neutralize the blood's acidity, and so makes the process far easier. If you should suffer from weariness, insomnia (loss of sleep) or a headache during this time it is only the result of the fast elimination process and will soon pass.

Upon rising. The juice of a fresh lemon in a glass of spring water. This should be served at room temperature.

Breakfast. A bunch of black grapes or a maximum of four apples, or a bowl of (sun-dried) fruit: apples, raisins, apricots etc; which have been soaked overnight in spring water.

Mid-morning. Herb tea (Rose hip, lemon verbena, chamomile, or lime blossom) or to your choice, with a teaspoonful of honey if desired, or a glass of spring water with the juice of a lemon.

Lunch. A glass of apple, pineapple or grape juice (ensure the juice is without preservatives). Plus half a fresh pineapple, or a bunch of black grapes or up to four apples.

Afternoon. Drink freely of herb teas, or apple, grape or pineapple juice, or spring water with fresh lemon juice.

Teatime. A bunch of black grapes or up to four apples.

Dinner. A bowl of fresh fruit salad (no limit on fruits or size of portion) with apple or grape juice as a dressing, or a whole fresh melon.

Evening. Drink freely of herb teas.

For the elderly, or those who will be working during this three day period, hot drinks of yeast extract can be taken between meals.

Replacement: days 4, 5 and 6

This part of the diet puts back what has been taken out of your system by stress. It begins by supplying an easily digestible protein in the form of yoghurt plus the mixed seeds rich in essential fatty acids. It also contains foods particularly rich in vitamins B_5 and B_3, the basic adrenal fuels for combating the effects of stress. B_3 also increases circulation and thereby helps to carry vital nutrients to the cells. Choline and inositol, well supplied in the granular lecithin, are also important in the replacement process.

First thing. The juice of a fresh lemon in a glass of spring water served at room temperature.

Breakfast. Up to 10 oz (¼ litre) of unsweetened natural plain yoghurt. One sliced banana, a handful of mixed sesame, pumpkin, and sunflower seeds, 2 tablespoons of wheatgerm and 2 tablespoon of lecithin granules.

OR

Soaked, mixed, dried fruits topped with unsweetened yoghurt, mixed seeds as before, plus wheatgerm and lecithin granules.

OR

Blend up to 10 oz (¼ litre) of natural (plain) unsweetened yoghurt with a banana, two tablespoons of lecithin granules and a dash of real vanilla essence.

Mid-morning. A glass of vegetable juice. (Fresh, carton or tinned.)

Lunch. Salad: choose from a mixture of lettuce, cucumber, green pepper, parsley, watercress, onion, celery, chinese leaves, spinach, chicory, cabbage, courgette, sprouted grains. Plus 3 oz (90g) of Ricotta or cottage cheese sprinkled with sesame, sunflower and pumpkin seeds.

Salad dressing for above: two tablespoons of cold-pressed olive oil, fresh lemon juice, garlic and herbs.

(Sesame, sunflower and pumpkin seeds can be chewed as a between meal snack.)

Afternoon. Drink freely of herb teas or vegetable juice.

Teatime.

Banana surprise:

Sliced banana with raisins, the three seeds and yoghurt.

OR

4 oz (120g) of sun-dried (not sulphur-dried) apricots.

Dinner. Salad as at lunch time. Jacket potato or brown rice, a little butter, no salt. (Optional) A glass of good red wine.

Rebuilding: days 7, 8 and 9

This part of the diet rebuilds your body. It contains foods such as mushrooms and fish and offal which are particularly rich in good quality essential fatty acids and proteins. It is also a bridge between the nine-day programme and a new way of eating which will help you maintain the benefits you have gained – a way of eating in which the acid/alkaline balance of foods is right, the intake of raw foods is high, and all the negative dietary factors such as coffee, ordinary tea, sugar and salt are eliminated.

Biochemic salt, which contains no sodium chloride, can be used in place of ordinary salt at this point in the diet, and can be purchased from most health food stores. It is particularly useful for those asthmatics who also suffer from high blood pressure.

First thing. Rose hip or lemon verbena tea with honey, or fresh lemon juice and spring water.

Breakfast. The Yoghurt Breakfast or soaked dried fruit breakfast or 2 eggs poached with a slice of rye or sesame crispbread, and a little butter. Herb tea or low tannin tea such as Earl Grey with lemon, or dandelion coffee.

Mid-morning. Drinks as at breakfast.

Lunch. Vegetable juice to drink.

Salad to be prepared as before but now tomatoes, raw mushrooms, radishes, small cauliflower florets, and fresh peas can be added. To the salad can be added 3 oz (90g) of any of the following: Ricotta, cottage, Gruyere, Emmental or any low fat, low salt cheese, or 3 oz of mixed nuts, almonds, brazils and cashews.

OR

A small grilled fish.

Teatime. Banana surprise or dried apricots or fresh melon.

Dinner.

Starter: Avocado with same dressing as for salad, or vegetable juice.

Main course: Salad with dressing and jacket potato or brown rice; grilled fish or fish roe OR free range chicken OR lamb's liver or lamb's kidneys OR a range of soft cheeses. A glass of good red wine (optional), herb tea, Earl Grey tea or dandelion coffee.

Summary of advice for intrinsic asthma

Foods to avoid
All dairy products such as milk, butter, and cheese. All products containing white flour and white sugar. All products containing listed 'E' numbers (see page 118).

Dairy produce should be avoided as it encourages the production of thick mucus in the throat and chest. White sugar and white flour products offer much less nutritional value than their 'whole' counterparts.

In place of butter there are some very good margarines to be found; low fat skimmed milk can also take the place of ordinary milk, and a range of cheeses can be bought which are made from skimmed milk.

For babies and young children with a milk allergy, goat's milk or sheep's milk can often be used instead.

Do remember the very basic rule is to maintain health and by doing so, avoid recurring chest infections, colds and flu. To achieve this you will need to ensure a healthy regular diet which contains plenty of salad, and fresh fish and meat in the summer months.

During the winter months special care must be taken with the diet: breakfast should be something cooked, either boiled eggs, or grilled bacon and tomatoes, or porridge oats. Plenty of warm drinks through the day, and a hot cooked meal later in the day. A regular supply of fresh meat, liver, poultry and fish, as well as plenty of fresh cooked vegetables and fresh fruit daily. The old-fashioned idea of keeping a stew on the stove through the winter months is worth keeping in mind for both young and old. There are a number of 'sweets' for children on the market which are made from wholegrains and honey, and contain no additives. Young children and elderly intrinsic asthma sufferers should also be taking a regular vitamin and mineral supplement throughout the winter months, as well as a daily dose of cod liver or halibut oil. This can be mixed with some fresh orange juice and shaken before drinking.

Summary of advice for extrinsic asthma

The extrinsic sufferer, on the other hand, will need to avoid the foods containing known allergens or substances which may stimulate the allergy reaction. This imposes a restriction on the number of foods available; because of this restriction care must be taken to ensure that a healthy diet is maintained.

As stated, many foods can now be purchased which are guaranteed free of additives or colourants. Despite this, all meat should be boiled before cooking and the water thrown away; this cleanses it from toxins and additives as well as rendering it more tasty.

The extrinsic sufferer must also learn to be firm when it comes to party and dinner invitations, and ensure that the host or hostess is aware of the restrictions regarding diet. If dining at a restaurant, it is wise also to ascertain beforehand that they would be willing to cook you something which will not cause a reaction.

In this way, with a little forward thinking, you can lead a reasonably normal life, and enjoy many of the delights the culinary world has to offer.

Children must be made responsible for their own asthma by teaching them to refuse those foods which they know will aggravate them. This includes sharing sweets, etc, at school. A list of foods which they cannot eat should be prepared for them to carry for reference, and to show other children as proof of their condition. If party invitations are received, a telephone call to the hostess explaining the allergy, will ensure your child is not given 'dangerous' foods. In this way mothers will be able to allow their children the freedom to attend birthday and Christmas parties without the fear of a sudden allergic attack.

The following food charts can be used as guide to the main sources of vitamins and minerals and should be used in conjunction with the different dietary suggestions.

Useful reading

E for Additives, by Maurice Hanssen (Thorsons).

Vitamins	Red meat	Poultry	Liver	Milk	Cheese	Butter/margarine	Eggs	Fish	Cereals and bread	Green vegetables	Root vegetables	Pulses/legumes	Nuts	Fruit	Other
Biotin			•				•				•	•			Especially peanuts. Cauliflower is good vegetable source.
Folic acid			•				•			•				•	Wheat germ and mushrooms are rich sources.
Niacin as nicotinic acid	•	•	•				•	•			•	•			Protein-rich foods such as milk and eggs contain tryptophan which can be converted to niacin in the body.
Pantothenic acid			•				•	•							Each food group contributes some pantothenic acid.
Pyridoxine	•	•	•				•	•	•						Especially white meat (chicken, fish) and whole-grain cereals.
Riboflavin			•	•	•		•		•		•	•		•	Found in most foods.
Thiamine	•		•					•			•	•			Brewer's yeast, wheat germ and bran are also good sources.
Vitamin A			•	•	•	•	•	•		•				•	Fish liver oil, dark green leafy vegetables such as spinach, and orange or yellow-orange vegetables and fruits such as carrots, apricots and peaches, are especially good sources of vitamin A.
Vitamin B$_{12}$	•		•	•	•		•	•							Obtained only from animal products.
Vitamin C										•				•	Especially citrus fruits, tomatoes, potatoes, broccoli, strawberries and melon.
Vitamin D			•				•								Dietary products are the best source, but the vitamin is also obtained by the body when the skin is exposed to sunlight.
Vitamin E			•			•	•		•	•				•	Vegetable oils, whole grain cereals and wheat germ are the best sources.
Vitamin K										•					Found in small amounts in fruits, seeds, root vegetables, dairy and meat products.

Charts taken from *The BMA Guide to Medicine and Drugs* courtesy of the publisher Dorling Kindersley Ltd.

Minerals	Red meat	Poultry	Liver	Milk	Cheese	Butter/margarine	Eggs	Fish	Cereals and bread	Green vegetables	Root vegetables	Pulses/legumes	Nuts	Fruit	Other	
Calcium				•	•				•		•	•	•			Dark green leafy vegetables, soya bean products and nuts are good non-dairy alternatives. Also present in 'hard' or alkaline water supplies.
Chromium	•				•			•	•							Especially unrefined whole grain cereals.
Copper	•	•	•					•	•	•		•	•			Especially shellfish, whole grain cereals and mushrooms.
Fluoride							•									Primarily obtained from fluoridated water supplies. Also in seafood and tea.
Iodine				•	•			•	•							Provided by 'iodized' table salt but adequate amounts can be obtained without using table salt from dairy products, saltwater fish and bread.
Iron	•	•	•				•	•	•	•						Especially liver, red meat and enriched or whole grains.
Magnesium				•				•	•	•		•	•			Dark green leafy vegetables such as spinach are rich sources. Also present in alkaline water supplies.
Potassium								•	•		•				•	Best sources are fruits and vegetables, especially oranges, bananas and potatoes.
Phosphorus	•	•	•	•	•	•	•	•	•	•	•	•	•	•	•	Common food additive. Large amounts found in some carbonated beverages
Selenium	•		•	•				•	•							Seafood is the richest source. Amounts in most foods are variable depending on soil where plants were grown and animals grazed.
Sodium	•	•	•	•	•	•	•	•	•	•	•	•	•	•	•	Sodium is present in all foods, especially table salt, processed foods, potato crisps, crackers, and pickled, cured or smoked meats, seafood and vegetables. Also present in 'softened' water.
Zinc	•						•	•				•				Sufficient amounts only in whole grain breads and cereals.

9
Other alternative therapies and asthma
Hypnosis

The use of hypnosis has been known for centuries and was used by the medicine men of ancient tribes to great effect in driving out the devils which they believed caused disease.

It was re-discovered in the 18th century by Franz Mesmer who began to use it in healing, but he was thought of as a quack by the doctors of those times and suffered professional ostracism because of his continued use of it. None the less, he claimed some remarkable cures in the so-called 'incurable' diseases of his time. He called it 'animal magnetism' and often employed 'stage props' and hand movements to induce a trance state. The use of hypnosis then began to fall into disrepute as more and more stage hypnotists appeared and hypnosis became associated with the music hall act.

The gradual return of hypnosis into its rightful role as a healing force is still finding opposition among many orthodox medical practitioners, but the word 'hypnotherapist' is now appearing more frequently on professional plates outside consulting rooms. Gone now are the stage effects favoured by Mesmer; instead the modern hypnotist often uses nothing more than a small pendulum or pocket torch, or modulated voice suggestions to induce the trance state.

The fear of hypnosis

A common fear is that of succumbing completely to the power of the hypnotist and being made, against our will, to reveal all those hidden secrets which we have locked away.

This is a difficult fear to allay, because there are varying reasons for the use of hypnosis, and a number of different ways of using it therapeutically. It must be admitted that one of the positive uses of the hypnotic trance is to help release suppressed pain or guilt which may be causing distressing symptoms on the surface. This is often achieved by the hypnotist exploring the subconscious mind until the cause of the symptom is discovered and removed. Only a complete trust in the hypnotherapist will overcome this fear.

Another common fear is that of not waking up from the trance state. To the best of my knowledge there is only one recorded case in which this happened and it involved the wife of a hypnotist. The hypnotist in question was in the habit of using his wife to try out different techniques of hypnotic induction and on this occasion when he attempted to wake her from the trance state she did not respond. In a panic he telephoned a hypnotherapist friend who immediately agreed to come to his house. Asking the husband to wait outside the room, the friend made contact with the hypnotized wife and asked why she did not wake up on the command. The wife responded by confessing that she believed her husband was having an affair with another woman, and this was her way of punishing him! While she was still in the hypnotic trance, the friend convinced her that she was genuinely mistaken, and on his command she then awoke.

Who can be hypnotized?

There is a popular belief that only weak-minded people can be hypnotized – in fact, the opposite is true. The more intelligent people make better subjects for hypnosis, whilst the mentally subnormal, young children, and very old people make the worst subjects. The reason is quite simple; during hypnosis the subject, guided by the hypnotist, is required to follow a single line of thought. The very young and the very old, and the mentally subnormal, are mostly incapable of concentration on this level as their mind tends to wander from subject, and they are easily distracted by the slightest outside influence.

However, there have been a number of times in my career when I have induced a deep trance both in old people and young children. On each occasion they were not aware that I was going to induce hypnosis and the method used in each case was invented at the moment of induction to suit the individual.

Case history of Mrs D
One particular case involved a lady in her seventies who was suffering from an incurable condition in her throat which prevented her from swallowing and from breathing properly. I was visiting her as a friend and I was very sad to see how quickly her condition had deteriorated in the few weeks since last I had seen her.

We sat talking across a bright fire one winter evening. She was finding it more and more difficult to get air as she talked, and eventually I suggested that she sat back in her chair and relaxed a little. I told her to look into the fire and her eyes would become heavy and close. When they closed I asked her if she could remember the happiest time in her life. She began to relax and a smile slowly spread over her face as she recalled an outing she had taken with some work friends to Blackpool. I asked her to take me there and she vividly recalled every aspect of that trip to me. Eventually I suggested that she took me to the beach and find a couple of deck-chairs in which we could rest. She was then told to visualize herself sitting in the deck-chair with the warm sea tickling around her toes. She was then told to go deeply asleep and to imagine that she was floating gently out to sea. She responded and slipped into a deep trance, during which I told her that when she awoke, all pain would be gone from her throat.

When she was awoken from the trance she recalled every moment and said it had been the nicest treat she could possibly have had to go back to Blackpool. A week later she died, without pain, and with a quiet tranquillity.

What will I experience in the trance state?

Most people who have experienced the trance state willingly volunteer for it again. They say that the feeling of utter relaxation, both mental and physical, is extremely pleasant, and one that is rarely experienced in the conscious state. Upon returning to normal, a feeling of well-being, of being recharged, alert and ready to go, and completely free of tension, are among the many comments I have heard over the years.

During the induction there are two main sensations experienced which seem to be evenly divided among subjects. The first is a sensation of heaviness in the body which increases through the induction until the subject is in deep trance; most people then lose awareness of the body.

The second is a pleasant sensation of lightness, of floating or drifting: these sensations are often so strong that I use them to deepen the trance state. For instance, if the patient is experiencing a sensation of lightness I will simply suggest that one or both arms are 'becoming extremely light'; in most cases the arms will then lift up of their own accord and the patient will enter a deep trance state.

The majority of people also remember the entire session clearly, both the induction and the therapy, when they awaken, and because of this some refuse to believe that they have been hypnotized.

This arises from a mistaken belief that hypnosis is a total state of unconsciousness, and that when you awaken it is as from a deep sleep. Were this true the hypnotist would lose touch with his subject both verbally and audibly, and the patient could not be woken unless he or she was perhaps shaken violently. This of course does not happen, the patient remains completely in touch with the hypnotist throughout the entire proceedings and is able to communicate at all times.

To avoid any misconception, the hypnotist should always explain before the induction what the subject should expect to feel and experience, as well as enquiring about special fears regarding hypnosis, as these may well prevent a successful trance taking place.

What is hypnosis?

This is a question that over the years has not been satisfactorily answered: Some claim that it is a state of sleep, whilst others say that it is state of hysteria. Neither would appear to be true. A sleep state implies that the person in a trance cannot hear you, as indeed in a normal deep sleep state we are mostly unaware of our surroundings, and yet in a hypnotic trance the subject can both hear and respond verbally to the hypnotist as in the case of the wife who would not wake up.

A state of hysteria would imply a highly nervous state, in which the subject could be liable to outbursts of high emotional activity, and yet the majority of people who undergo successful hypnosis are rational, calm people, often highly intelligent, and will experience a total recall of the entire hypnotic state.

My personal explanation from years of observation of the hypnotic trance is that a reversal of the conscious and subconscious takes place temporarily, under the guidance of the hypnotist.

This reversal is brought about by holding the attention of the conscious mind for a short time, while suggestions are fed to the subconscious which will induce a deeply relaxed mental state, as well as a state of heightened awareness. This at first appears to be a paradox, but there is no doubt that if you question somebody who has experienced the hypnotic trance they will tell you that they were extremely aware, whilst at the same time they appeared to be drifting a long distance away.

Although the basic trance state remains the same, it can be used in a number of different ways therapeutically: the three methods most used are *regressive hypnosis*, *post-hypnotic suggestion* and *direct suggestion*.

In the chapter on stress control the roles of the conscious and subconscious minds were explained, and how impressions and memories stored in the subconscious are often be triggered by a stimulus from the conscious level. The triggering of these memory switches by outside stimulus can sometimes result in unwanted reactions.

Regressive hypnosis

Case history of Miss X

I often recall the case of Miss X, a woman in her mid-twenties who had risen to the position of personal secretary to a company director. She was suffering from an uncontrollable tight feeling in the chest; so violent was this feeling at times that she found it almost impossible to breathe and was unable to carry out her professional duties.

The tight feeling had commenced with a slight catching of the breath approximately six months earlier. Her doctor was puzzled and had referred her to a specialist at her local hospital. Tests had not revealed any pathological cause, and her doctor had prescribed tranquillizers, but with little effect. It was decided to attempt regressive hypnosis: this is when a person is taken back in time by the hypnotist who is looking for a possible trigger which may have caused the surface symptoms. It was not until she had regressed to the age of three years that the trigger was spotted. She was brought up by very strict 'Victorian' parents and they lived in a large Victorian house. Her father had a large study in which none of the children was ever allowed. At the age of three she remembered wandering through the house and, seeing the door to the study open, she went in. A drawer in the desk was open, and she went to it and put her hand inside; at that moment her father appeared in the doorway and roared in anger to see her at his desk. She, being very frightened, caught her breath and then ran shaking from the room. During the regression her breathing became very tight, and it was noted that the difficulty in breathing had commenced at work following a trivial incident. Her boss was out, and she urgently needed a special file from the drawer of his desk. Entering his office, as was her privilege as his personal secretary, she had gone to the drawer when he suddenly returned, and jokingly, in order to make her jump, had demanded from the doorway 'what the blazes do you think you are doing?'. From that moment her breathing had tightened and gradually worsened. Under hypnosis it was explained to her that the two incidents were linked, and that her boss's feeble joke had awakened the fear of her father, and her subconscious memory had then begun to associate her father and her boss as one. She was told that it was this subconscious fear linked to the incident in her father's study and the office that was causing the tight chest. She was then awoken from the hypnotic trance and her breathing from that time returned to normal.

Regressive hypnosis offers a valuable method of exploring those regions of the subconscious mind that are normally inaccessible. It has been said that we never forget anything, that everything we see, hear, smell, taste or feel, is stored away in our subconscious. But because the subconscious has no discriminating power it stores painful as well as pleasant memories, and because we avoid dwelling on painful memories we store them in deep and often inaccessible places of the memory. If the memory is one of emotional pain or guilt then some time in the future it will need resolving. If it is not resolved, one of its ways of reminding us of its presence, even though we have seemingly forgotten it, is by producing surface symptoms.

These often bear no resemblance to the problem and can vary from irrational behaviour patterns to extreme mood swings, or irritability or depression. Sometimes physical symptoms of feeling 'uptight' can manifest, which are of particular interest when treating nervous asthma.

I have known suppressed guilt to cause a complete nervous breakdown. These symptoms are often treated by a doctor with an antidepressant drug, and although it will keep the symptoms quiet for a time, it can be as dangerous as hiding a suppurating wound under a bandage until it has turned gangrenous and the part has then to be amputated.

The skilled use of regressive hypnosis can be likened to the surgeon's knife cutting away the bad part and allowing clean new tissue to form.

Post-hypnotic suggestion

The triggering of memory switches by an outside stimulus can cause unwanted symptoms but it can also result in beneficial reactions, and hypnosis uses this in a positive way.

The method of triggering these switches is called *post-hypnotic suggestion* and relies upon the ability of the subconscious mind to obey commands in the 'walking state' that have been placed during the hypnotic trance. It is similar in some respect to the exercises mentioned in Chapter 4 on 'stress control' where by repeating a set

mental exercise the subconscious mind is slowly programmed to react in a positive way to situations that used
to cause a negative reaction.

Post-hypnotic suggestion can bypass this slow program-
ming if needed, and place the trigger immediately.

Case history of Mr B

Mr B was a retired naval officer who, until he had left the
sea and taken a job in the City, had never experienced an
asthma attack in his life. The peculiarity of the case was
that whenever he took a holiday by the sea his asthma
completely disappeared, but in the City he needed frequent doses of his inhaler to breathe. Under hypnosis he
was told that whenever he felt an asthma spasm beginning, he would take a slow deep breath and remember
the rolling sea and open skies and experience a complete
freedom of breathing. Three sessions of post-hypnotic
suggestion completely cleared his asthma attacks, and
several years later he reported a total cure.

How can hypnosis help asthma?

It should be understood that, like any other therapy,
hypnosis will only help when its use is definitely indicated: it is not a cure for every asthmatic. Nevertheless,
there are cases when hypnosis will offer considerable
help, as already illustrated in the previous case histories.

Nervous asthma

When the asthma has a definite nervous origin and is
worsened from anxiety or fear, hypnosis can offer positive
help in a number of ways.

Under direct suggestion the subject is told that in place
of the weakness there is a positive feeling of strength,
which will enable the sufferer to overcome such things as
shyness, anxiety, fear, etc.

Hypnosis can also offer assistance with the use of post-
hypnotic suggestion, which will activate a positive subconscious command that will help overcome the situations
which stimulate asthma attacks.

They hypnotherapist may in some cases decide on the
use of regressive hypnosis if a hidden cause is suspected
to the fear or anxiety which is promoting the asthma.

Extrinsic asthma

We know that the cause of extrinsic asthma lies in the body's reaction to an allergen which produces asthma. Hypnosis may be used in several different ways to help this form of asthma: firstly, by direct suggestion it may be possible in some people to promote the body to become less sensitive to specific allergens. It may also be possible through post-hypnotic suggestion to lessen the effect of the allergen on the body. It is acknowledged that after a number of attacks caused by known allergens, the subconscious mind prepares in advance the way it will trigger the body to react, in this situation hypnosis may help by deprogramming the subconscious mind in order to lessen the strength of the reaction to the allergen.

There is no doubt that the mind has a powerful effect on the body. For instance, under hypnosis a subject can be touched with a wooden pencil on the arm and told that the pencil is a red hot poker. Not only will the hypnotized subject recoil violently from the pencil, but you will often see a red weal appear on the skin, and sometimes a blister.

Intrinsic asthma

Stress and tension, both physical and mental, due to prolonged difficulty in breathing may be relieved in the intrinsic asthmatic by relaxation under hypnosis.

The breathing difficulties experienced can also be helped by placing a 'trigger' in the subconscious which will enable the asthmatic in some instances to control the asthma spasm without the use of an inhaler.

Difficulty with sleeping at night due to breathing problems, in both young and old, may be helped by post-hypnotic suggestion which is often accompanied by a better quality of sleep than usual.

For the young instrinsic sufferer at school, hypnosis has been used with good results in promoting a positive attitude toward schoolwork, sports, and life in general.

Hypnosis can also be useful for those who cannot manage the visualization/relaxation techniques. Using the trance state, the hypnotist can implant a physical trigger (such as slow deep breathing) which will automatically activate a release of tension in the breathing pattern and produce a feeling of mental relaxation whenever it is used.

Osteopathy

Osteopathy is a system of physical medicine which specializes in correcting minor bone displacements by manipulation. The philosophy of osteopathy follows the basic premise of holistic medicine that 'complete health cannot exist unless the body is in complete harmony'. The minor displacement of a bone can give rise to pain and impede the flow of the 'vital force'; when this happens because the body is not in perfect alignment dis-harmony prevails.

When viewed alongside the other therapies outlined in this book, the asthmatic may well be forgiven for asking what benefits a system of physical medicine could possibly offer for a lung condition?

The first answer must be that if you are attempting to stimulate the healing power in the body to produce a cure, a state of harmony must exist, and osteopathy assists the body to achieve this by removing any impediment that may be causing discomfort or pain.

The second reason is because a minor displacement can cause pressure on related nerves, and in some instances this can produce symptoms of tight chest and restriction of breathing. It has been proved beyond doubt that by treating certain displacements, symptoms of asthma can be relieved in some cases. The most common displacements that affect the asthmatic take place in the spine. The spine consists of a number of bones called vertebrae: there are 24 moveable vertebrae and 9 fixed vertebrae in the spine. The fixed vertebrae are at the base of the spine and form the two areas known as the sacrum (the wedge-shaped bone on which the spine sits), and the coccyx (or tail bone).

The moveable vertebrae consist of 7 cervical or neck bones, 12 thoracic vertebrae which are situated between the base of the neck and the pelvis, and 5 lumbar vertebrae which are those in the low back which appear to give the most trouble to the average person.

Between each of the moveable vertebrae is a disc or pad which acts as a shock absorber. Through the centre of the spine runs the spinal cord, similar to the wiring loom of a motor car, with nerves leading to different muscle groups and organs of the body. A slight displacement of a vertebra can produce pressure on one of these nerves and cause symptoms which vary from slight to acute pain, or even paralysis of a limb or limbs.

Thoracic displacements

The thoracic area, which encompasses the ribcage and the area of the spine which supports the ribs, is the most likely place for the asthmatic to experience trouble. Small displacements in this area, caused by the bent back stance, or prolonged coughing, can cause pressure on nerves which directly affect the chest. The symptoms can range from slight discomfort to great restriction in the ability to take a deep breath. Also because of a closely related nerve, symptoms can be experienced in the heart area, and these can vary from pain to palpitations (a fast and audible thudding of the heart).

Muscular problems

Alongside these bony displacements can often be found related conditions in the muscles caused by the abnormal strain arising from the displacement. Osteopathy recognizes these strains or imbalances which, if left untreated, will often lead to related conditions in the soft tissue of the body, namely in the muscle fibre which in turn may itself produce symptoms of pain. This can have a long-term lowering effect on the health and well-being of the individual.

Soft tissue manipulation

As well as joint manipulation, osteopathy has a method of dealing with these soft tissue conditions called 'soft tissue manipulation'. This is a form of specialized massage, based on the 'Swedish massage technique', which assists in breaking down adhesions in the soft tissue, and restores blood supply and elasticity to the muscle.

This can be of particular value to the asthmatic, as one of the most common muscular conditions experienced by the asthmatic is tightness in the neck and shoulders, caused mainly by the hunched stance adopted through difficult breathing. A condition known as *fibrosis* is formed by tiny granules which set between the muscle fibres and eventually form layers of adhesion which prevent the fibres from expanding and contracting in their normal way. Sometimes these adhesions cause inflammation of the muscle fibres, and the condition is then known as fibrositis, which is a distressing and painful condition producing a gnawing ache in the muscle with restriction of movement.

The symptoms of fibrositis are generally better from movement and warmth, and worse from rest or becoming chilled.

The condition in the neck and shoulders can slowly worsen if untreated and cause vertigo (giddiness), and eventually chronic tiredness and an inability to concentrate, or a feeling as if the head was 'full of cotton wool'.

Following osteopathic treatment the asthmatic will often experience greater ease in standing erect, which in turn means there is less pressure on the chest, and the bonus is easier breathing.

Low back pain and asthma

Of the osteopathic causes of low back pain, the most common are lumbar disc strain, and strain of the sacro-iliac joint – this is the area of the pelvis in wich the sacrum (the wedge-shaped bone) fits between the two wings (iliacs) of the pelvis.

Any displacement in the low back usually produces pressure on a nerve, and the pain causes the patient to protect the area, which in turn produces a slight tilt of the pelvis.

This produces a deviation in the alignment of the shoulder girdle, causing one shoulder to drop and the other to lift. The subsequent tilt of the body causes the spine to describe an 'S' bend, and at the centre of the bend are the thoracic vertebrae. The pressure at the centre of the 'S' will often cause one of the thoracic vertebrae to slightly displace, causing the symptoms already explained.

The asthmatic with a history of low back pain would be wise to have the condition treated, especially if the asthma appears to have worsened since the back pain began.

Many asthmatics find that an annual visit to their osteopath for thoracic manipulation and massage results in improvement to their breathing.

The Alexander technique

This is a system of teaching an awareness of posture: it does not seek to provide physical treatment. Its practitioners are highly trained and usually require a series of visits in which the patient's professional and home environment is studied, and then training is given in awareness and correction of postural faults. The technique can provide improvements in poise and breathing, as well as reducing mental and physical tensions.

Acupuncture

This is a system of medicine originated in China some thousands of years ago, in which tiny needles are placed at specific points of the body to stimulate the 'healing force'. Its philosophy is that the essential healing power, known as *chi*, flows along the lines of *meridians* in the body. These lines, which are negative or positive, or *yin* and *yang*, follow certain channels in the body, which can be blocked by emotional, physical or spiritual causes. The insertion of the acupuncture needles at very specific points provide a stimulus which aids in clearing the blockage and restoring the lines of harmony along the meridian channels.

The philosophy of acupuncture is very much in harmony with the philosophies underlying the other 'natural therapies' in holistic medicine, and many asthmatics claim improvement in both their asthma and their general health from its application.

Aromatherapy

This is a therapy which employs the use of massage with essential oils to produce a relief of symptoms in numerous conditions. The quality of the oils used is important, together with the expertise in blending them for use in treating specific conditions. It follows very closely the knowledge and use of aromatic and stimulating, as well as relaxing and warming oils employed in herbal medicine. For the asthmatic, great relief can be obtained both from the antiseptic and the expectorant and relaxing properties of these essential oils when used in conjunction with the correct massage techniques.

Reflexology

This is a system of treatment which seeks to treat disease by working on certain pressure points mainly situated in the soles of the feet. It follows a similar philosophy to that of acupuncture but restricts the pressure points on which it places importance. Its practitioners employ massage and pressure to specific areas of the sole of the foot according to the condition being treated. Many patients have reported improvement to their asthma condition from such treatment.

This system of pressure points is also employed for diagnosing the cause of disease.

The Bach remedies

This is a system of treatment devised in 1933 by Dr Edward Bach, a Harley Street specialist in vaccine immunity. He decided to specialize in treating the effects rather than the cause of disease by using a combination of homoeopathic and herbal remedies. He reasoned that as a result of the disease, the patient suffered mental symptoms that in turn had a lowering effect on the 'vital force', and that by relieving these symptoms the body would be released to fight off the disease.

He therefore experimented and eventually produced a list of extracts from plants, flowers and trees, and prepared them homoeopathically to be specifically employed in treating the mental/emotional symptoms of the patient, regardless of the disease. He claimed many cures with his remedies, and today a total of 38 different extracts, each with the mental/emotional symptoms clearly defined, is available from health stores and herbal dispensaries. The tonic effects of the single or combined extracts on the asthmatic can be very beneficial, and a special combination of those extracts called the *Rescue Remedy*, taken in the form of drops on the tongue, can provide quick relief to the effects of an asthma attack.

10
Factors within the environment

Our environment at the present time is a very delicate issue, and the subject of much discussion and concern, as governments worldwide try to tackle the ecological problems caused by humanity. Many people believe that environmental pollution may be the cause of some diseases as well as hyperactivity in children and aggression in adults.

It is known that contamination from lead can produce learning difficulties and behavioural problems in children, and recently Southampton University claimed to have found a link between aluminium and Alzheimer's disease (senile dementia). There are some toxic metals which are known to have a detrimental effect on asthma and we shall be exploring them later in this chapter, but the most common, and probably the most troublesome pollution for both forms of asthma is smog. Not the solid blanket-type smogs that at one time enveloped our towns and cities and could bring traffic to a grinding halt: those are a thing of the past due to government intervention with such legislation as the 'Clean Air Act'. In some respects they were far easier for the asthmatic to deal with because if smog was about, you just didn't venture out. But in this present day the smogs, or polluted air, are not so easily detected, and because of this they present a greater danger to the asthmatic, who may be subtly and slowly affected over many months. Many asthmatics live in heavily populated areas, or work in areas of intense industrial activity; in both of these environments, the air can be heavily polluted with soot and chemicals as well as vehicle exhaust. Each produces its own type of smog: that from industrial pollution is known as industrial smog, and that arising from cities is known as photochemical smog, which arises from high density exhaust fumes and inadequate sunlight.

Asthma in its various forms is a highly sensitive disease, which means that it can be easily brought on by outside stimulus. The asthmatic needs to examine his or her environment seriously and identify the factors which could aggravate or cause the condition. The possible factors are numerous and not all are easily identifiable, so it is hoped that the following general categories will be a guide.

Environmental pollution

Industry

The sources of industrial pollution are almost too many to mention, but the most important are the industrial wastes which are discharged on to the earth, and into our air and water. These do eventually have some effect on all of us to one degree or another. The effects are often too subtle to relate to poisoning from pollution, but sometimes a sensitive condition such as asthma will quickly respond, especially to airborne pollution. Industrial chemical waste often finds its way into our drinking water, and a number of the nitrates and some toxic minerals are not filtered out through the normal cleansing processes.

Also remember that our drinking water contains chemicals which have been used for processing and cleaning the water – aluminium is one that was recently highlighted.

Toxic smoke from factory chimneys can be a particular hazard especially for the intrinsic asthmatic, causing wheezing and shortness of breath when it is breathed in. It may also contain chemical allergens that could trigger extrinsic asthma.

We also get the results of this type of pollution in another way when it returns as acid rain to pollute the soil and rivers, and eventually enters our drinking water.

We allow discharges from nuclear power plants, both into the sea and air, and although we have been assured this is harmless, and does not exceed the permitted limits of pollution, we are receiving disturbing reports that the incidence of blood disorders has shown a significant increase in the areas in which they are sited. It would be interesting to know if there has been any significant increase in asthma in a fifty-mile radius around such stations.

With regard to those asthmatics who work in industrial environments, UK government legislation which came into force on October 1st 1989 gives the Health and Safety Executive the power to force employers to protect employees who may suffer from the effects of the following industrial pollutants: chemicals; solvents; dusts; fumes; gases; oils; cleaning agents and micro-organisms.

This law comes under the 'Control of Substances Hazardous to Health Regulations' and further information can be obtained from the Health and Safety Executive, Unit 5–9, Grain Industrial Estate, Harlow Street, Liverpool L8 4UH.

This is of particular importance to those asthmatics who suffer aggravation to their condition from any of the aforementioned industrial pollutants, as employers are now required under law to provide essential protection if you are affected by them.

Food industry

Pollution in this category does include some additives in our food known to cause or aggravate extrinsic asthma. Details of these were listed in the chapter on food. A number of fruits such as apples and citrus fruits receive a wax spray to preserve and heighten the shine and colour of the fruit in order to make it more appealing to the undiscerning public. This spray may be proved to contain undesirable elements, not so easily washed off the fruit by reason of the wax coating.

Dyes and tenderizers used in the preparation of fresh meat to heighten colour and texture, in order to make it more appealing to the consumer should also be questioned, especially by extrinsic sufferers because of the potential 'E' numbers which of course will not be listed as on a pre-packed food item. Whilst the intrinsic sufferer should also be questioning the purchase of this treated product in relation to the quality of their food and general health.

The present controversial use of irradiation to extend the shelf life of a range of food products may not prove to be of as much benefit to the consumer as it is to the producers and retailers.

Farming

Farms and farmers are also being blamed for their part in promoting environmental pollution. Long gone is the image of the healthy life related to the country air and home-cooked fresh food. The tearing up of hedgerows to make larger fields which can easily be managed by one man and a giant tractor is causing an ecologic imbalance of nature. The birds and insects which kept the crop pests under control have reduced in numbers, and in their place the farmer must use chemical sprays to ensure his crop is not destroyed by the creatures of nature. The earth has no time to rest between crops any more, because sound business practice means a continuous production, and in order to achieve this the ground must be 'false fed' with chemicals in order to provide nutrients for the growing crops.

Farm animals are mostly kept in strictly controlled atmospheres in order to obtain the maximum size of animal. Hormones are injected into them to promote growth and control the quality of the meat. Consequently among the farming discharges which are excreted through animal waste, we now have hormones as well as nitrates, as well as the chemicals which have been used to kill weeds and insects all being either washed into streams and rivers or allowed to soak through the earth into the water table, and eventually into our drinking water.

The feeding of foodstuffs to some animals and poultry which contain the remains of other dead animals, has recently come to light through outbreaks of food poisoning and animal diseases such as BSE or 'mad cow disease'. These practices may present a hazard to the allergic asthmatic as well as to the intrinsic asthmatic.

Smoke from stubble burning which contains traces of the toxic compounds used in the sprays and fertilizers, can also present problems to both types of asthma, and is often to be found many miles from its source if the weather conditions are right.

The public

The public, who are becoming vociferous in their complaints regarding industrial and farming pollution, should themselves look at the pollutants they release into their environment.

These include vehicle exhaust fumes, with or without lead, which release deadly toxins into the atmosphere. This can be demonstrated in any town when one has to frequently stop breathing for a few seconds as some bus or lorry roars by spewing thick clouds of exhaust toward pedestrians. A traffic jam can also present a problem for the asthmatic, whether travelling on foot or in a vehicle, due to the buildup of fumes in one area from exhausts. Emissions from household fires, as well as gas fired central heating boilers or oil fired boilers, also add their toxins to our atmosphere and make breathing for the asthmatic that much more difficult.

We produce sewage waste in such large quantities that it must be diverted into rivers and seas. It too contains toxins and bacteria as well as hormones which are not easily broken down by nature, and like the farm waste, it eventually finds its way back into our water.

The asthmatic who undertakes to run the hazard of smoking tobacco in any form is responsible not only for promoting his own condition, but also causing breathing problems for those around him, whilst those who do not have asthma should consider the asthmatic when lighting up in public places. It goes without saying that the asthmatic should avoid those places where a heavy atmosphere of tobacco smoke prevails.

Aerosol gases from numerous sources including spray polishes, anti-perspirants, and deodorants, could also cause breathing problems if sprayed in the vicinity of the asthmatic, and both intrinsic and extrinsic sufferers should avoid the use of them, for the sake of their condition as well as the delicate condition of the earth's atmospheric protection layer.

The list of environmental pollutants that may have a detrimental effect on the lungs and the general health is frightening both to intrinsic and extrinsic asthmatics.

And yet the asthmatic can lead a reasonably symptom-free life by taking certain positive actions to cope with these potentially asthma-causing environmental pollutants.

The first step toward action is to ascertain which pollutants cause your asthma symptoms.

Extrinsic or allergic asthma

Let us deal first with allergic asthma. The first step is to identify the allergens which affect you; in some cases this is quite simple, as the reaction is always immediate to one or more easily identifiable substances. In some cases, however, the allergic reaction can be delayed for a few hours or a day, and in these cases the task becomes more difficult. Over the years a number of different allergy tests have been devised which help to identify which allergens affect you. In some cases this enables desensitizing treatment to be given in order to render the patient immune from further reaction.

The following allergy testing methods are a sample only of those available at the present time. Always seek the advice of a qualified practitioner as to which is most suitable for you.

Allergy testing methods

Vega testing
This is an electrical device which uses the known acupuncture points to measure the electrical response of a patient to allergens which are introduced into the circuit of the machine. It is painless, and simply involves the patient grasping a small electrode, whilst another electrode held by the person testing is gently applied to selected points on the surface of the body. It can be used for testing for allergy reaction to foods as well as chemicals.

Skin testing for allergies
Most people are familiar with skin testing, which is carried out by injecting tiny amounts of substances suspected of being allergens just under the surface of the skin. Instead of injecting, some practitioners use a scratch testing method – this is when the substance being tested is applied to a small scratch made on the skin. The

test response is the same in both methods: if the person is allergic, the skin responds by producing a swelling in the area of the injection, and this generally indicates a degree of allergy is present to the substance being tested.

An interesting phenomenon which has been noted is that in some cases when there has been no reaction to the applied allergen, that a diluted amount of allergen used does produce a positive reaction. This may support the claims of homoeopathy that the diluted dose is often more effective than the crude.

Although quite effective, skin testing does have its dangers, as there have been cases when the reaction to the injected allergen was sudden and produced a severe asthma attack.

Applied kinesiology

This test relies in changes of muscle strength being detected during the time that a small amount of allergen is placed under the subject's tongue, or held in the hand.

The person being tested is asked to stand and extend an arm with the palm of the hand uppermost. The person testing then gently exerts pressure downwards on the extended arm and measures the power of the muscle resistance. Then the same pressure is exerted again, but this time with a sample of the allergen either on the extended hand, or placed under the tongue. If the person is allergic to the substance a definite weakening in the resistance of the arm muscles is detected.

Elimination diet

This is one of the older methods of allergy testing, and relies on the patient undergoing a fast for a set period, usually five to seven days. At the end of the fast period the patient is given one food only at the first meal, at subsequent meals a different food is given until the entire range of foods that the patient had been eating is tested. The foods to which the patient shows an allergy reaction are then withdrawn from the patient's diet.

This method does have disadvantages: it is time-consuming, it can be weakening, and it does not allow for the interaction of two or more foods causing the allergy.

Radiesthesia or pendulum testing for allergies

Dowsing is a term which many associate with hazel twigs and water, but the science of dowsing has advanced a great deal. The modern dowser uses a pendulum, and prefers to use the term *radiesthesia* in place of dowsing. Its use is no longer restricted to finding underground water: I know of architects who use a pendulum to find deep drains, or hidden water pipes. Oil companies sometimes employ dowsers to advise them where to drill, and now the pendulum has entered the clinic, and is used both for diagnosing and prescribing.

Some practitioners of the pendulum need only a body chart with the patient's name written on it to test for allergic substances. Others test each substance with the patient holding a sample of the substance: the reaction of the pendulum when held above the patient will reveal a positive or negative reaction, and from this the operator can diagnose the existence of an allergic reaction.

As most people have some ability to use a pendulum, allergy testing can be carried out by yourself at home. *The Practical Pendulum Book* by D. Jurriaanse, published by The Aquarian Press, provides both instruction on the use of the pendulum as well as numerous charts for different tests.

Blood testing for allergies

Radio allergo sorbent test

This is a method used by doctors for testing for antibodies in the blood in relation to specific foods. It is meant to show, by the presence of specific antibodies to specific foods, that an allergy to that food exists.

There has recently been some doubt as to the reliability of this testing method.

Cytotoxic testing

This method is claimed to be 80 per cent accurate, and works by exposing white blood cells to suspected allergens. Physical changes in the white cells take place if an allergen is present, and these changes can be detected by an expert and a diagnosis formed.

Hair analysis

This cannot be classified as a means of allergy testing, but it can provide a useful source of information regarding mineral levels in the body, and this includes toxic minerals.

In a previous chapter the importance of the major minerals was explained, and how a lack of them could undermine the body's health. Hair analysis also reveals if you have too much of a specific mineral in the body, which in some instances can be as undesirable as having too little. The levels of some minerals can also be an indication of trouble elsewhere in the mineral balance, and in some instances if above or below the normal range can interfere with the absorption of other minerals or vitamins. This may have an adverse effect in both types of asthma as the intrinsic sufferer needs to ensure the correct balance of minerals in order to promote a healthy constitution, whilst an imbalance in one or more minerals to the extrinsic sufferer may promote a greater sensitivity to allergens than normal. Most laboratories check across a range of minerals which are normally shown on an easily readable chart, with maximum and minimum levels shown as a guide. This form of testing also usually checks for excessive levels of poisonous minerals such as mercury, lead, aluminium, arsenic, and cadmium, as these can have a damaging effect on the body. For instance high levels of aluminium can adversely affect the nervous system, and cause a drying of the mucous membranes with symptoms of hoarseness, dry cough, wheezing and constriction of the chest. These symptoms would be called 'pseudo asthma' in a non-asthma sufferer, but were these symptoms to be experienced by an asthmatic as an aggravation to their existing asthma it could prove dangerous. Cadmium, arsenic and mercury can also produce a number of symptoms in the chest which would cause difficulty in breathing.

Asthmatic symptoms produced by toxic metals

Aluminium
- Dryness of mucous membranes.
- Cough starts soon after waking in morning.
- Hoarseness, with wheezing, rattling respiration.
- Chest feels constricted, talking aggravates.

Other symptoms:
- Staggers on walking. Heels feel numb.
- Dry sore throat. Feeling as if something lodged in throat.

Arsenicum Alb.
- Unable to lie down for fear of suffocation.
- Asthma which is worse at midnight.
- Darting pain through upper third of right lung.
- Suffocative catarrh with cough which is worse after midnight.
- Dry cough as from irritating fumes after drinking.

Other symptoms:
- Extreme tiredness. Very restless at night.
- Gradual loss of weight. Much anxiety.
- Sneezing without relief. Cannot bear sight or smell of food.

Cadmium
- Interrupted breathing during sleep.
- Chest feels enlarged. Asthma symptoms worse squatting.
- Cough with loss of consciousness.

Other symptoms:
- Burning and cutting pain in the stomach.
- Intense feeling of sickness.
- Obstruction of the nose with swelling.

Mercury
- Cough with yellow expectoration.
- Cannot lie on right side during asthma.
- Asthma worse at night and from warmth of bed.
- Stitching pain from right lower lung through to the back.

Other symptoms:
- Frequent cold sweats all over.
- Weakness and shaking in legs and arms.
- Chronic tiredness and trembling.
- Foul smell from the body.

Case history of Mr B

Mr B consulted me with an unsual problem. Each year around April or May he would commence symptoms of depression, chronic tiredness, and extreme restriction in breathing. These symptoms would persist until September, when they disappeared as mysteriously as they had come. His doctor was puzzled and ordered blood tests and chest x-rays but these proved negative. He had been experiencing the symptoms for four years when he consulted me and was relying on antidepressant and antihistamine drugs for six months of the year. Several different therapies were tried, without success. The great difficulty was that I could only treat him during the six months that he was experiencing the symptoms; when they cleared we would have to wait for six months for them to reappear. It was during the winter months, when he had no symptoms, that I decided to have a hair analysis report on him prepared. A sample of his hair was sent to the laboratories and when the report came back it showed that he had a major lack of most of the essential minerals; it also showed a level of arsenic in the sample which was above the accepted safety level. Mr B had no idea where he may have ingested arsenic: his job, an office executive, was not situated near any chemical plant, and he had not been eating excessive amounts of parsley, a plant known to contain higher levels of arsenic than other plants.

A mineral supplement was given to make up the mineral deficiencies and high doses of vitamin C and garlic were prescribed to help the body overcome the arsenic. We waited expectantly for April/May to arrive. It did, and so did his depression, tiredness and breathing problems! I decided in the light of the hair analysis report to prescribe Arsen. Alb. in the 200th potency to act as an antidote. It worked, and within a week he was feeling normal without the use of his drugs. However, each time I withdrew the homoeopathic Arsen. Alb., his symptoms returned. I was puzzled, and questioned him extensively on his dietary, business and social habits, seeking a possible clue to his recurring symptoms. The only digression from his normal habits around April/May time was that he walked to work instead of taking his car or the bus. He lived on the edge of the country, and enjoyed watching the trees and fields burst into green. He showed me his walking route, which skirted around two farms before arriving on the edge of town where his office was situated. On investigation it transpired that both farmers were in the habit of spraying young crops through the period of months that Mr B experienced his symptoms. The evidence appeared to favour the crop spraying as the source of arsenic contamination. Two further hair analyses at six-month intervals showed the high arsenic levels had completely gone, although Mr B still needs his arsenic antidote each April/May.

The weather

So far we have dealt with the allergic and non-allergic asthma triggers relating to our environment arising from pollution and additives to our foods. There is however one major environmental factor which is capable of affecting both types of asthma and that is the weather.

Intrinsic asthma

There appears to be a very definite relationship between the symptoms of intrinsic asthma and the prevailing weather conditions at different times of the year. Cold, dry air seems to aggravate many sufferers' symptoms, causing a narrowing of the airways, as well as promoting the conditions favourable to upper respiratory infection, especially if the body temperature is allowed to fall. The intrinsic asthmatic should take particular care to wear warm clothing in such conditions.

Equally, high humidity when the weather is warm and damp, can promote difficult breathing conditions, and some asthmatics experience hyperventilation, which is breathing in and out more air than they need, which causes a feeling of oxygen starvation. This feeling is not necessarily an asthma attack, but it may promote one because of its 'knock-on' effect.

Warm, dry atmospheres appear to suit intrinsic asthma sufferers, but even then, if the barometer is falling, it could signal the approach of increasing humidity or storm conditions, which may promote difficult breathing conditions. Also, a windless day may allow an increase in the smog effect in built-up areas, and cause aggravation to the asthmatic.

The intrinsic sufferer should also be aware of sudden changes in the weather. The most dangerous are when the weather suddenly changes from warm to cold and the body temperature is allowed to drop. This and getting wet through can set up the ideal conditions for chest infections which can lead to asthma.

Extrinsic asthma

The weather can play a vital part in the symptoms of the extrinsic asthma sufferer. Wind can affect the distribution of pollens and mould spores and concentrate them in a particular area, and during the summer months most local radio stations provide a service of regular broadcasts through the day giving the pollen count in your area.

Rainy conditions can hold down pollen and wind-carried irritants, and give periods of relief to the allergic sufferer; unfortunately, damp humid conditions also promote the growth of such spores, and can hold pollen in a concentration which presents dangers to the extrinsic sufferer.

It is very important in the proper management of asthma for the asthmatic to know the type of asthma that they have, and also to understand and recognize the triggers which will promote an attack. Only then can you plan to take the appropriate preventative action.

Preventative action plan

Be wise!

If you have been prescribed medication by your doctor, follow his or her instructions regarding the dosage and frequency of your drugs, and if prescribed carry your inhaler at all times, especially if you have no asthma symptoms as this is the time in which you are likely to forget, and you may suddenly need it!

If you are under treatment from an alternative medicine practitioner ensure that you carry your emergency remedies, if prescribed, at all times.

Do remember that all of the suggestions contained in this book are designed to be followed *alongside the current drugs* you are taking. Should you experience improvement in your symptoms, only stop your drugs under the guidance of your doctor.

The following ideas are useful tips for both forms of asthma as they assist you to control some of the environmental factors in *air and water* which play a part in causing asthma symptoms.

Water filters

Not to be confused with water softeners, which are designed to produce soft water *which should not be drunk*.

Water filters come in a number of designs and sizes. The most common are the jug filters, which contain 1 or 2 pints/½–1 litre. They are fitted with a renewable filter which should be changed regularly according to the manufacturer's instruction. The filter usually contains a mixture of ion exchange resin and activated carbon which between them reduce hardness in the water as well as levels of lead, copper, chlorine compounds and free chlorine. They are available from most health food shops and super- and hypermarkets.

There are a number of more sophisticated water filtering systems which vary from small metal canisters fitted direct to the incoming drinking water pipe, usually under the sink, to large tank systems which filter the tap water to entire buildings. These normally contain a silver filter which also removes chalk, lead, copper, chlorine compounds and chlorine. The advantage against the jug system is that you have a continuous flow of filtered water both for drinking and cooking. The manufacturers of both types of filter claim that using filtered water stops kettles from 'furring up' and tea and coffee tastes better and leaves no scum around the cup. The disadvantages of this

kind are that they cost a lot more, and the filter must be
changed after approximately one to two years (according
to the quality and quantity of water you use).

Peak flow meters

The breathing capacity of both forms of asthma seems to
diminish before an asthma attack, but this is not always
outwardly detectable. Now a meter has been designed
for measuring lung capacity, which is light and easy to
carry. This enables the asthmatic to detect diminished
breathing ability and provides a degree of warning that
they are becoming vulnerable to an attack. This is a
valuable aid for asthmatics, especially children, who
should be taught to use it before and during prolonged
physical activity. Its use may prevent them reaching a
dangerous breathing crisis. It should also heighten their
enjoyment of life and provide them with more confidence
in their ability to manage their own asthma. It could be
equally useful for adults, for by taking a daily lung
capacity reading an accurate graph can be built of
environmental conditions such as weather or stress
which cause a worsening of their condition and allow
timely preventative action. The Peak Flow Meter can be
obtained from some chemists or ordered direct from
Clement Clarke International Ltd, 15 Wigmore Street,
London W1H 9LA. (Tel: 071-409 1062.)

De-humidifiers

The quality of air, as we have already discussed, is very
important to both the extrinsic and the intrinsic asthmatic,
as both find that extremes of damp and dry air can cause
aggravation.

Aggravation from damp air outside can normally be
prevented by covering the mouth with a scarf, but a damp
atmosphere in the home is not always recognized as a
possible cause or aggravation of asthma. Some houses are
damp because of faulty construction, others through lack
of proper heating which causes condensation in the winter
months, and some through bad ventilation when not
enough 'through air' is allowed in a room.

Any of these causes can promote humid conditions,
which are easily identified by windows streaming with

condensation, or black mould spores on the walls of a room, particularly behind furniture or in cold corners. Heavy cigarette smoking in confined spaces such as a small low-ceilinged room, or a car, can cause high humidity. The symptoms of humidity are to cause irritative coughing as tiny particles of moisture adhere to the tiny hair triggers in the nose, throat, and lungs. Breathing can feel tight with wheezing and the desire for an open window.

The obvious solution is to identify and correct the cause, but if this is not possible then it would be wise to consider a method of de-humidifying the atmosphere.

The simplest and cheapest method to achieve this is by using *silica gel*, which has the ability to absorb considerably more than its own volume of water. The silica-gel dehumidifier is usually a plastic container about the size of an average sandwich box. It can be square or round, and is divided into top and bottom by a central shelf with numerous holes in it. The silica gel is placed on the shelf, and the water it collects from the atmosphere is in turn collected in the base of the container. According to the size of the room, you would need between one and three to a room. The silica gel does need renewing from time to time.

There are varying other types of de-humidifier on the market, usually much larger and more sophisticated, often requiring a source of electrical power. The cost of these varies enormously, from several hundred pounds upward.

Humidifiers

Humid air conditions as previously described are mostly associated with older houses. However, the modern sophisticated houses with their efficient double glazing and central heating systems cause the opposite conditions, dry air. This to the asthmatic also presents problems, as lack of some humidity in the air can dry out your air passages, and cause a buildup of static electricity in the house which is bad news to the extrinsic sufferer. The answer to the problem of dry air is very simple and inexpensive: a saucer of water placed near a radiator in

each room is all that is required. The heat causes the water
to evaporate slowly into the room which provides a small
amount of moisture in the air, sufficient to overcome the
problem.

Some retailers sell small receptacles for water, designed to
be hooked over the radiator: again, these are inexpensive
and overcome the possibility of an adult foot landing in
the saucer or worse, an inquisitive baby.
  Asthmatics who live in such atmospheres would be
wise to always ensure that the house is properly humidi-
fied, and especially the bedroom at night.

There are more sophisticated humidifiers available; the
latest from Mountain Breeze Products uses ultrasonic
sound vibrations to break water into a fine mist which
they claim allows a far greater efficiency in the absorption
of the particles into the air.

Ionizers

We are surrounded by ions, or electrically charged mol-
ecules of carbon dioxide, nitrogen and oxygen. They are
either positively or negatively charged. The number of
positive or negative ions around us at any one time is
reliant on environmental factors. For instance, more negative ions are to be found by the sea, or on mountain tops,
and on open moorlands. A greater number of positive
ions are to be found in houses, cars, offices; city streets
where there is a high level of traffic smog; just before a
thunderstorm, as well as in the vicinity of television sets
and computer screens, or where there is a high density of
working electrical equipment.
  An awareness of the effect of positive and negative ions
is important to both extrinsic and intrinsic asthmatics, as
one brings benefit and the other brings aggravation.

Positive ions
The effect of a high concentration of positive ions on the
average person was researched by Professor Kreuger of
the University of California. He found that positive ions
stimulate the body to produce a hormone called *serotonin*.
The effect of high levels of this hormone on our system is

to cause difficulty in sleeping, tiredness and listlessness, as well as depression. It is important for both extrinsic and intrinsic asthmatics to realize the effect of the ions in the atmosphere around them, because when there is a predominance of positive ions the extrinsic asthmatic will find a marked increase in the number of airborne allergens, such as dust particles, pollens, spores, and soot. The intrinsic sufferer may well find that he/she doesn't feel so good, breathing is not so easy as it could be, and the allergens which affect the extrinsic asthmatic may well cause the intrinsic asthmatic a tightening of the airways, if they concentrate in large enough numbers.

Carpets, curtains, blankets and sheets as well as wallpaper in the average home can be producers of positive ions. The bedroom especially can be highly charged throughout the night, whilst just walking across the average sitting room which is positively charged will produce clouds of small particles of dust, fibres, and pollens.

Most modern motor cars present the same danger of positive ions to the asthmatic: the seat covers, the carpets, the metal bodywork, and the electrics all produce positive ions. The extrinsic asthmatic could be sitting daily in a box of potential aggravation without realizing it.

Negative ions
These are produced naturally where there is sharply moving water, that is why sitting by the sea or a tumbling mountain stream makes us feel good. The air feels clean and alive. This is because the negative ions attach themselves to dust, pollen and small particles in the air, the dust becomes charged and is attracted to the nearest neutral surface. So you could look upon negative ions as air cleansers which not only clear the air of pollens, etc, but also smoke and, some say, bacteria.

It therefore follows that the asthmatic must benefit from being in an atmosphere that has more negative ions, and this factor should be considered when deciding a holiday venue.

Meanwhile, for those who are not going on holiday, if you live or work in an atmosphere that produces positive ions you can buy a small piece of modern technology called an ionizer. An ionizer produces a constant stream of negative ions, and is small enough to be placed by your bed, or on your desk, and you can even buy one that works from the cigarette lighter in the car.

There is no overdose possible of negative ions, and manufacturers claim a reduction in colds, asthma, and bronchitis in a significant proportion of users of ionizers.

Children's asthma card

The Asthma Society provides a strong support for asthmatics. It has over twenty pamphlets explaining varying aspects and treatment of asthma. The Asthma Society and The Asthma Research Council will soon merge to become The National Asthma Campaign. As a result of National Asthma Week, held in October 1989, a children's Asthma Card was launched. The cards are issued by your doctor and they give details of treatment, how to deal with a serious attack, the name, address and telephone number of the family doctor and the hospital consultant. A copy will be kept by the child's family and the school.

Smog help line

In response to recent heavy smog buildup as a result of increased traffic on the roads and the hot weather, the National Asthma Campaign has announced its intention to man a twenty-four-hour emergency telephone help line. The service will be in action for the next three years. Watch the national press for details or telephone The National Asthma Campaign.

Resources

Useful books

Worries and Fears [in children], Dr John Pearce (Thorsons, 1989).

Herbal Stress Control, David Hoffmann (Thorsons, 1989).

Staying Ahead, John Wareham (Thorsons, 1989).

Protection for Life, Dr Yukie Niwa and Maurice Hanssen (Thorsons, 1989).

Vegetarian Children, Sharon Yntema (Thorsons, 1989).

Successful Fasting, Dr Hellmut Lutzner (Thorsons, 1990).

Change Your Life – Right Now, Dr Sidney B. Simon (Thorsons, 1989).

Open to Suggestion, Robert Temple (The Aquarian Press, 1989).

Green Pharmacy, Barbara Griggs (Jill Norman and Hobhouse, 1982).

Potter's New Cyclopaedia of Botanical Drugs and Preparations, R.C. Wren (C.W. Daniel, 1988).

The Vitamin Bible, Earl Mindell (Arlington Books, 1985).

E for Additives, Maurice Hanssen (Thorsons, 1987).

Diets to Help Hay Fever and Asthma, Roger Newman Turner (Thorsons, 1989).

Homoeopathic Medicine, Trevor Smith (Thorsons, 1982).

Homoeopathy: the Family Handbook, (The Homoeopathic Development Foundation Ltd) (Unwin, 1987).

Bach Flower Therapy, Mechthild Scheffer (Thorsons, 1986).

Yoga Self-Taught, Andre van Lysebeth (Allen and Unwin, 1978).

Index

genetic weaknesses 16–17
gonorrhoea miasm 16, 17
gravity, change in, and night
    time symptoms 9

habit patterns 44–5
    relaxation trigger 46
habits 42, 44–5
    see also habit patterns
Hahnemann, Dr Samuel 16, 73–4
hair analysis 156, 158–9
hairspray 15
happiness, from positive thought
    34
health, personal level 21
heart beat, harmonizing with
    breathing 48–9
heartburn 28
herbal medicines 15, 20, 22,
    58–72
    asthma treatment 62–7, 69
    case histories 70–2
    pharmacopoeia 63–7
    specific remedies 68–9
histamine 12
holidays 26–7, 36, 85–6, 164, 166
home environment, asthma cause
    25–6, 36, 162–5
    prevention techniques 55–6
homoeopathy 15, 22, 73–92, 154
    materia medica 86–92
house dust mite 13
house dust *see* dust, in home
houseplants 25, 26
housewives, and asthma 85
humidifiers 163–4
hypnosis 133–42
    case-histories 134, 135, 137–8,
        140
    induction by counting method
        53
    post-hypnotic suggestion
        139–40
    regressive 137–9
    trance state 135–6

IgE antibodies 12
immune system 11–12, 94, 114–15
industry, pollution irritants 13,
    23, 149–50

influenza *see* flu
infusions 59–60
intrinsic asthma 12, 13, 15
    aerosols avoidance 152
    case histories 72, 121–2
    environmental factors 149
    food additives 150–1
    food needs 22, 129
    and holidays 26–7
    and humidity indoors 162–4
    hypnosis treatment 141–2
    induced by physical activity 24
    late onset 29
    and positive and negative ions
        164–6
    tissue salts treatment 109–11,
        114–15
    vitamin/mineral supplements
        94
    weather effects 159–60
iodine 104, 105, 132
ionizers 25, 164–6
iron 104, 105, 106, 132
Isoprenaline 18

kinesiology, applied 154
Kreuger, Professor 164

lifestyle, positive changes 35–7
lungs 10, 47, 49

magnesium 104, 105–6, 132
mast cell stabilizers 17–19
mast cells 12
mediators (body chemicals) 12
medical insurance, and travel
    abroad 27
mental changes 37
mental relaxation *see* relaxation
    techniques, mental
Mesmer, Franz 133
metabolism 94–5
metals, toxic *see* toxic metals
miasms 16–17
mind *see* conscious mind; control,
    of asthma, through the
    mind; subconscious mind
mineral salts 108–16
minerals 93–4, 104–16
    chelated 107

in elderly 30, 31
prevention 22, 28
relaxation trigger 46
subliminal 39–42
and vitamin deficiency 95
and work environment 23
subconscious mind 43, 44–5
and development of physical
habits 41
and hypnosis 137, 139–40
post-hypnotic suggestion
139–40
success
cause of stress 39, 40
from positive thought 34, 38
summer, allergies 9, 80
Swedish massage technique 143
sympathomimetics (drugs) 18
symptoms 9–10

Ten Steps Guide 123
Theophylline 19
thinking *see* positive thinking
thoracic displacements 143, 144–5
thought *see* positive thinking
tissue salts 108–16
toxic metals 156
asthma symptoms 157–8
case histories 158–9
toys 25
trace elements 108–16
trachea 10
trigger, for relaxation 46
post-hypnotic suggestion
139–40, 141–2
on visualized walk 50, 51, 52
trigger factors, for asthma attack
160
tubercular miasm 16, 17

vapour bath 69
Vega testing 153
vehicle exhaust fumes 152
visualization 49–53
Vitamin 'A' 98, 99, 131

Vitamin 'B' complex 97, 98,
99–101, 131
Vitamin 'C' 97, 98, 100, 101–2,
105, 120, 131
Vitamin 'D' 95, 97, 98, 102, 104,
106, 131
Vitamin 'E' 98, 102–3, 131
Vitamin 'K' 95, 98, 103, 131
Vitamin 'P' 103
vitamin/mineral supplements
20–1, 22, 107–8, 129
during pregnancy 28, 29, 37
vitamins 93–103
for asthma 97–8
deficiency factors 95–7
food chart 131
uses 98
see also vitamin/mineral
supplements

walks, visualized 50–3
water filters 161–2
weakness, constitutional *see*
constitutional weakness
weather conditions 10, 13, 15,
113–14, 159–60
weight problems 22
wheezing 10, 29, 30
reason for 11, 13
whooping cough 83–4
winter, aggravations 9
precautions 76–9
work, attitude to 32–3, 35, 36–7,
40
work environment, asthma cause
22–3
prevention techniques 56–7,
150

xanthines (drugs) 18, 19

yeast spores 14
yoga breathing 46–7, 53

zinc 104, 106–7, 132

Of further interest . . .

THE ALLERGY HANDBOOK
The Essential Guide to Successful Treatment
Dr Keith Mumby

Do you suffer from Asthma? Eczema? Mouth Ulcers? Catarrh? Do you often experience Panic Attacks? Insomnia? Irritability? Mood Swings?

These are just some of the symptoms associated with allergy.

In this excellent, bestselling book, Dr Keith Mumby, 'the allergy detective', draws on his long experience of treating allergic reactions to foods and environmental pollutants to offer clear, practical advice on how to recognize allergic reactions and what you can do to combat them – the natural way.

It includes information on:

- the role of elimination diets
- the links between nutrition and allergy
- different methods of allergy testing
- where to go for specialist advice

Fully revised and updated it includes special sections on:

Candida Albicans • Post Viral Fatigue Syndrome • Electro-magnetic medicine • Food allergies • Environmental medicine

This book is quite simply essential reading for anyone interested in the alternatives to traditional medical treatments.

Dr Keith Mumby is a medical doctor who has achieved renown for his successful treatment of many thousands of sufferers at his Food and Environmental Allergy Clinics.

CHILDHOOD ASTHMA
A Complete Treatment Plan
Dr Mike Whiteside

Asthma – difficulty in breathing caused by the constriction of the airways in the lungs – is a very frightening and unpleasant condition. For parents, the sight of their asthmatic child struggling for breath is particularly distressing; however, this positive and innovative book will provide new hope and much comfort for all parents of asthmatic children.

Written by a general practitioner with three asthmatic children of his own, as well as years of experience treating young asthma sufferers in his practice, CHILDHOOD ASTHMA offers an enormous range of practical, detailed information and advice on the management of asthma in children, including:

- the nature of asthma, its cause and symptoms
- common asthma tests
- prevention using inhaled medication and alternative therapies
- correct use of inhalers
- the role of the body's immune system
- the role of allergens
- the treatment of attacks, both mild and severe
- treatment using alternative therapies, including breathing exercises, homoeopathy, acupuncture and self-hypnosis

Written in a clear and authoritative style, with numerous illustrations, CHILDHOOD ASTHMA is an indispensable book for any household with an asthmatic child.

THE ALLERGY HANDBOOK	0 7225 1657 6	£4.99	☐
CHILDHOOD ASTHMA	0 7225 2245 2	£5.99	☐
HOW TO BEAT HAYFEVER	0 7225 2829 9	£4.99	☐
NEW SELF-HELP ASTHMA & HAYFEVER	0 7225 1899 4	£2.99	☐
DIETS TO HELP ASTHMA & HAYFEVER	0 7225 1933 8	£2.99	☐
ASTHMA & ECZEMA SPECIAL DIET			
COOKBOOK	0 7225 1821 8	£4.99	☐
SUPERHEALTH	0 7225 2589 3	£9.99	☐

All these books are available from your local bookseller or can be ordered direct from the publishers.

To order direct just tick the titles you want and fill in the form below:

Name: _____

Address: _____

_____

_____ Postcode: _____

Send to: Thorsons Mail Order, Dept 3, HarperCollins*Publishers*, Westerhill Road, Bishopbriggs, Glasgow G64 2QT.
Please enclose a cheque or postal order or your authority to debit your Visa/Access account —

Credit card no: _____

Expiry date: _____

Signature: _____

— to the value of the cover price plus:
UK & BFPO: Add £1.00 for the first book and 25p for each additional book ordered.
Overseas orders including Eire: Please add £2.95 service charge. Books will be sent by surface mail but quotes for airmail despatches will be given on request.

24 HOUR TELEPHONE ORDERING SERVICE FOR ACCESS/VISA CARDHOLDERS — TEL: **041 772 2281.**